LIVING WITH EPILEPSY

Living with Epilepsy

A guide to taking control

**DR PETER FENWICK
AND ELIZABETH FENWICK**

BLOOMSBURY

Extract from *Women and Epilepsy*, Edited by M.R. Trimble (1991)
reproduced by permission of John Wiley and Sons Ltd.

First published 1996 by Bloomsbury Publishing Plc, 2 Soho Square,
London W1V 6HB

Copyright © 1996 Dr Elizabeth and Dr Peter Fenwick

The moral right of the authors has been asserted

A copy of the CIP entry for this book is available from the British Library

ISBN 0 7475 2340 1

10 9 8 7 6 5 4 3 2 1

Typeset by Hewer Text Composition Services, Edinburgh
Printed in Great Britain by Cox & Wyman Ltd, Reading

CONTENTS

1 What is epilepsy?   1
● What is epilepsy? ● Types of seizure ● Who has
epilepsy? ● Common causes of epilepsy ● What is
it like to have a seizure? ● Myths about epilepsy

2 Diagnosing epilepsy   25
● What to do for a first fit ● Referral to a
specialist ● Special investigations

3 Treating epilepsy   40
● The modern treatment of epilepsy ● Drug
treatment ● First-line drugs ● Second-line drugs
● State-of-the-art drugs ● You and your doctor
● Becoming fit free ● Outlook

4 Surgery for epilepsy   62
● Temporal lobe surgery ● Frontal lobe surgery
● Hemispherectomy ● Callostomy ● The right age
to operate

5 Alternative approaches to seizure control   75
● Biofeedback ● Relaxation ● Covert desensitization
● Psychotherapy ● Videorecording ● Aromatherapy
● Acupuncture ● Meditation ● Yoga

6 Controlling your own seizures   93
● Learning about your seizures ● Looking for links
● Finding a counter measure ● Making seizures
happen

7 **Non-epileptic seizures**   103
   ● Confusion about diagnosis ● Treating non-epileptic seizures

8 **Living with epilepsy**   111
   ● Taking control of your life ● Happiness – a good anticonvulsant ● Diet ● Alcohol ● Photosensitive epilepsy ● Safety precautions ● When a parent has epilepsy ● Aid in an emergency

9 **Epilepsy, employment and the law**   136
   ● Driving regulations ● Epilepsy and employment

10 **Children with epilepsy**   143
   ● Diagnosing children ● Helping the child with epilepsy ● Epilepsy at school ● Practical safety tips ● Parents' concerns ● The adolescent ● Recreational drugs ● Advice on future employment ● Sexuality

11 **When epilepsy becomes a handicap**   173
   ● Children with learning disabilities ● Some rare disabling conditions ● Employment opportunities

12 **Sex, pregnancy and epilepsy**   184
   ● Marriage ● Sexual side-effects of epilepsy ● Women ● Pregnancy ● Breast feeding and baby care

13 **Postscript**   200

Appendix A: Glossary   201

Appendix B: Useful Addresses   207

Index   211

1

What is Epilepsy?

This book is about epilepsy. Perhaps you are reading it because you have epilepsy yourself, or because a friend or family member has developed it. If you have just discovered that epilepsy affects someone close to you, you may feel very apprehensive about what the future holds. Epilepsy can seem frightening to anyone who knows little about it but I hope that this book will show you that it need not either rule or ruin your life. People who have epilepsy are ordinary people who lead ordinary lives. This is how one such person first discovered that she had epilepsy:

Jennifer was a normal, healthy young woman enjoying her first year away at college. Enjoying it so much, she had to admit, that studying had not been a real priority and her first year exams that week had been rather stressful. Still, they were over, and now she could relax. She had been up most of the night dancing at an end of term ball, and now, with her boyfriend Michael, she was walking to a pleasant riverside pub to meet some friends for lunch.

Suddenly she was overcome by the weirdest feeling. She wasn't sure that she could stand and had to sit down. 'What's the matter? Are you OK?' Michael asked, but Jennifer couldn't explain what the matter was. 'I just feel really funny,' was the best she could do. 'It's hot and you're tired and probably hungover. No pub lunch for you — I'm taking you home,'

Michael said firmly. 'Have an early night and we'll see how you are tomorrow.'

The next day Jennifer still felt exhausted, and didn't want to go out. But then she seemed to recover and as it was near the end of term and she had no more 'funny turns' she forgot about it.

It was about two months later, when she was home from college on vacation, that she had her first big attack. It was late, she was very tired but decided to make herself a cup of tea before going to bed. She was sitting on a kitchen stool drinking her tea when she suddenly felt herself falling backwards. She heard a crash and then nothing more until she recovered consciousness on the floor with her mother bending over her.

Jennifer's terrified parents called an ambulance and in the hospital emergency department Jennifer was told that she had had a seizure. There was no need to keep her in, the casualty officer told them, but Jennifer should make an appointment with her GP who would explain everything to them. Jennifer felt almost too shocked to speak, but she managed to ask the casualty officer the question which was uppermost in her mind. 'Of course you won't have to leave University,' he reassured her. 'Probably you'll have to take medication to stop any more seizures. But I can see no reason why you shouldn't go back to college next term and finish your course.'

Epilepsy is one of the oldest disorders known to man and, until very recently, it was one of the most misunderstood. Imagine a friend, someone you know to be normal and sane, suddenly falling down in front of you, jerking in a terrifying way and then lying as still as death. And if you found this frightening, how would you feel when, as if by some miracle, they seemed to arise from the dead, in full possession of their senses once more and apparently none the worse for what had happened? It is easy to understand why the ancient Greeks called epilepsy the 'sacred disease', and why in biblical times someone having an epileptic fit was thought to be possessed by the devil.

Hippocrates himself was one of the first people to try to change people's attitudes towards epilepsy. He recognized that damage on one side of the brain caused convulsions which started on the opposite side of the body and tried to persuade people that the disorder was due to natural rather than supernatural causes. Unfortunately science, as so often happens, proved less attractive than superstition. Epilepsy retained the power both to frighten and to mystify. There were no real advances either in the understanding of epilepsy or in its treatment until near the end of the nineteenth century, and myths and misconceptions about the disorder continued to plague sufferers until almost the present day.

What is epilepsy?

Epilepsy is not a disease. It is not a mental illness. The word (from the Greek) literally means 'to take hold of or seize'. To have epilepsy is to have recurrent seizures (or fits or convulsions – they all mean the same thing). And a seizure is a temporary state of abnormal electrical activity within the brain. Note the word temporary – it is important. People with epilepsy sometimes have occasional seizures, but they do not have an illness any more than someone who has occasional headaches.

The brain is one of the most complex organs in the galaxy. It consists of over ten million million neurones, each connected to about 6,000 other neurones. When the brain is functioning normally, myriads of neurones fire (that is, give out a burst of electrical energy) transmitting information from cell to cell. This whole process continues 24 hours a day and is responsible for our emotions, feelings, understanding, movements and behaviour – in fact everything we think or feel or do.

What is amazing is that most of the time the system works so well – the processes are always carried out correctly. Sometimes, however, the brain becomes too excitable. This can happen because it is damaged, or because of an inherited genetic tendency to excitability. This super-excitability occasionally leads to areas of the brain going out of control with many cells firing together. Sometimes cells in the surrounding area are drawn into the process and start to fire abnormally too. These discharges – bursts of abnormal electrical firing – last from seconds to minutes and then the brain returns to its normal functioning state. While the discharge lasts it causes a temporary change in our emotions, consciousness, intellect or behaviour. This is known as a seizure.

Anyone can have a seizure under certain conditions. In fact, fits are very common; one person in 20 will have a major fit during their life, but two-thirds of people who have a single fit never have another. The brain can become temporarily more excitable than normal during drug or alcohol withdrawal, and so people who are trying to 'dry out' or to withdraw from drugs are quite likely to have seizures, but only under these conditions. Seizures may follow extreme sleep deprivation or prolonged hunger too, because these conditions make the brain temporarily more excitable, so that it occasionally produces the sudden burst of electrical firing that leads to a seizure.

Children's brains are more excitable than those of adults, so children are always more seizure-prone. Some babies and young children also have an inherited tendency to have seizures when they are running a high temperature, but this does not mean that they have or will develop epilepsy (see febrile convulsions, p.155). The fact that you have one fit does not mean that you have epilepsy any more than one swallow makes a summer. You won't be regarded as suffering from epilepsy unless your fits recur.

The usual yardstick for a diagnosis of epilepsy to be considered is for two fits with no obvious cause (such as drug withdrawal or a high fever) to occur within two years. This definition of epilepsy – two fits within two years – also means that epilepsy is by no means a life-long sentence. Many people outgrow their epilepsy, and if you have had a two year period free from fits you will be regarded as no longer suffering from epilepsy. However, once you have had epilepsy, there is always a small chance that your fits may recur at a later date, because you don't necessarily lose the tendency to have fits.

WHAT HAPPENS DURING A SEIZURE?

Most people's view of a typical epileptic fit is the major *grand mal* seizure in which the sufferer falls to the ground unconscious and jerking. But this is only one of the very many different types of seizure. A few people suffer from more than one kind of seizure, and the form their epilepsy takes may change, so that they may have different kinds of seizures at different stages of their life. To understand exactly what happens during the different kinds of seizure, and why they occur, we need to look a little more closely at the way the brain works.

Information is transferred within the brain in the form of electrical impulses, passed from cell to cell by chemical messengers, which can make the cells which transfer information either more or less excitable. As each brain cell 'fires', it stimulates a neighbouring cell and this in turn fires and excites the next cell along the pathway. Some of the cells which fire are inhibitory cells and these tend to damp down the activity, so that it does not run rampant through the brain, out of control.

How excitable the brain is depends on the balance of those chemical messengers which excite and those which inhibit cell firing. In some people the brain cells are more excitable than normal. They will fire more easily and, instead of the normal damping down by inhibitory cells, there is a sudden paroxysmal burst of electrical activity within a group or groups of cells. This is known as the 'epileptic spike discharge' and its presence can usually be picked up through the scalp by use of the EEG (see p.31). However, even if you have these spike discharges they needn't cause any disturbance and you will normally be quite unaware of them. It is only when the damping down activity fails more extensively that the abnormal activity spreads. Whole areas of cells become involved and start to fire in these paroxysmal bursts: a seizure (convulsion or fit) then occurs.

Sometimes, if there is an area of localized brain damage, the cells at the centre of this damaged area are so altered that they can no longer fire normally. These cells are called pacemaker cells, and they fire abnormally and continuously. Nothing stops them. However, they do not, of course, cause fits continuously. Something else must happen to make a seizure occur.

We know that before a seizure occurs the pacemaker cells all clump together and discharge in unison. As they clump together, the pacemaker cells recruit the cells surrounding the damaged area into the discharge and it is this spreading of the discharge which causes a localized or focal seizure. Yet why should this happen in the first place? What makes the pacemaker cells which are firing all the time suddenly interest the cells surrounding them in their faulty messages? The answer seems to be that some change in behaviour or thinking, or even something as simple as drowsiness, makes these neighbouring cells temporarily more excitable so that they can be drawn into the seizure discharge more easily.

These focal seizures can sometimes spread to include the whole brain – a process called secondary generalization, which often results in a major seizure (tonic clonic convulsion, see p.7).

Types of seizure

The kind of seizure you have will depend on which part and how much of the brain is affected, and how widely and rapidly the seizure spreads from its point of origin.

WE CAN DIVIDE SEIZURES INTO TWO TYPES:

Generalized Seizures arise over a wide area of the brain and affect both sides of the body right from the start of the seizure.

Partial Seizures arise only in a limited area of the brain and so may only have a limited effect on the mind or the body. Partial seizures used to be called focal seizures because they arise from a focus, an area of damaged tissue, sometimes a small scar in the brain.

Partial seizures may be either simple, which means that consciousness is not altered during the seizure, or complex, which means that the seizure spreads out from its point of origin into areas of the brain which are responsible for maintaining or constructing consciousness.

GENERALIZED SEIZURES

The tonic clonic (*grand mal*) seizure

The generalized tonic clonic seizure is the best known and the most common type of generalized seizure. It is everyone's idea of a typical epileptic fit – what used to be called the *grand mal* seizure. *Grand mal* is still the name by which many people know them best, but people who have epilepsy and work with it now always call these seizures 'tonic clonic' and so this is the term I shall use in this book.

During a tonic clonic attack the person falls to the ground unconscious. In the first 'tonic' phase of the attack the muscles of the body contract, the arms and legs go straight and rigid, the mouth clenches tight and the whole body is stiff. The seizure may end at this point, or it may continue with a second, 'clonic' phase during which the muscles of the body jerk in unison, starting at a rate of about once a second, slowing to a rate of once every four to six seconds, and then stopping. Sometimes a convulsion consists only of this jerking phase. At the end of the seizure the muscles relax. Sometimes, but not always, bowel and bladder control are lost during the fit. If you suffer from tonic-clonic seizures you will probably find that the extent of the two phases of the fit will vary from time to time.

Usually these seizures occur quite suddenly, out of the blue, though a few people do have a vague feeling of being unwell for a few seconds immediately before a seizure. But if you suffer from *grand mal* seizures you will not experience any 'aura' or odd sensation at the beginning of an attack to warn you that it is about to occur.

Absence seizures

Another very different kind of generalized seizure is the 'absence' (what used to be called the *petit mal* seizure). In fact 'absence' describes this kind of seizure very well, and so this is the name which I shall use for these seizures throughout the book. During an absence the person – nearly always a child – has a 'blank' period from seconds up to half a minute or so long during which they are usually quite unaware of anything that is happening to them, though they may rarely retain a dim awareness of what is going on around them. They may look pale, and their eyes are fixed and glazed. Sometimes their head will slump forward, though usually they will stay in the same position they were in before the attack. There may be brief muscular twitches around the eyes, or jerks of the limbs, but because this is a generalized seizure, affecting the whole brain, these movements will always be symmetrical, and always affect both sides of the body. When the attack is over, the child will carry on exactly as before, as if nothing has happened, continuing with whatever they were doing or saying when they were interrupted. Usually about five or ten such attacks will occur in the course of a day, but sometimes runs of attacks occur in rapid succession.

To the onlooker it may look as though the child is simply day-dreaming or not concentrating, and the attacks may even pass quite unnoticed as there are virtually no after-effects. However, an EEG recording (see p.31) made during one of these absences will reveal a characteristic pattern, called spike and wave. The good news about absence seizures is that they usually disappear around adolescence, though occasionally they'll persist into adulthood or give way to tonic clonic seizures. But while they are occurring they can be very disruptive of a child's education, as well as giving him or her an undeserved reputation for inattentiveness. So it is important that they are diagnosed, and that they are treated.

A few children have more complex absence seizures, which last rather longer and are accompanied by lip-smacking, chewing or fumbling movements, but the EEG still has the same characteristic spike and wave pattern.

Myoclonic epilepsy

These are sudden, very brief and uncontrollable muscle jerks which usually arise from a focus on one side of the brain, affect only one side of the body, but can be generalized and affect both sides. They look essentially the same as the myoclonic jerks which most people occasionally experience just as they are dropping off to sleep. The person may be flung off balance, or if they are holding something it may be dropped or thrown violently away.

Juvenile myoclonic epilepsy

Juvenile myoclonic epilepsy (JME) is a common generalized epilepsy, with a significant genetic component. The first seizure usually occurs in the teens, most frequently between the ages of 13 and 15. For some months or years before the first seizure, the person often has mild myoclonic jerks – the involuntary sudden jerky movements of the limbs that everyone experiences now and again, usually when they are dropping off to sleep. These jerks are usually in one or both arms, and occur within an hour of waking. In a few children the myoclonic jerks are preceded by mild absence seizures which start around the age of ten.

Seizures are triggered by lack of sleep and alcohol. About half the children who have JME are photosensitive, and for them flashing lights are a potent seizure trigger (see p.108–9).

The outlook is good for children with JME. Up to 90 per cent become seizure-free with medication (usually sodium valproate). Unfortunately if medication is withdrawn there is a high relapse rate, even for someone who has been seizure-free for several years.

> *Sixteen-year-old John was used to his mother getting irritated with him at breakfast. He was always clumsy and jittery first thing in the morning; often his arm would jerk as he was trying to drink, and coffee would go everywhere. But no one took it seriously until one Sunday morning John had his first tonic clonic seizure on waking. The night before he'd been at a party, had got home at 1 a.m. and tumbled into bed exhausted and, in his own words 'well tanked up'. Later, when John and his parents were talking to their doctor, John wouldn't even have thought to mention his early morning jitteriness if the doctor hadn't specifically asked him if he ever had any twitchiness in his limbs first thing in the morning.*

Drop attacks

Drop attacks affect all ages and consist of a sudden, very brief loss of consciousness and muscle tone, so that the person does, literally, drop to the ground. The real danger of these attacks is that they occur quite without warning, and so the person may be badly bruised or hurt.

Infantile spasms (West's syndrome)

One of the most serious kinds of childhood epilepsy is also, fortunately, one of the rarest. A few infants develop what are called infantile spasms between the ages of about three months and a year. The spasms – sudden, massive contractions of all the body muscles – occur because the normal activity of the brain is disturbed, and this can happen for a variety of reasons. As they grow older many of these babies do, sadly, have learning difficulties or develop autisms, and many continue to have seizures.

SIMPLE PARTIAL (OR FOCAL) SEIZURES

Partial seizures are always caused by damage to some part of the brain, and always begin in that area of the brain, though they may later spread. If you have partial seizures you will nearly always have some kind of 'aura', a feeling or sensation that you will come to recognize at the beginning of your seizure and that acts as a warning to you that the seizure has begun. The aura is caused by the start and early spread of the electrical discharge within the brain.

The characteristics of the aura will depend on the part of the brain involved. That is why when your doctor is making the diagnosis he or she will want to know in as much detail as possible the feelings or symptoms you experience at the start of the seizure. If your seizure starts in the motor cortex (the part of the brain that controls movement), your aura will probably consist of a movement of part of the body, usually a thumb or the face, perhaps an arm, hand or foot.

A common form of motor epilepsy is Jacksonian epilepsy, named after the English neurologist Hughlings Jackson, who lived at the turn of the century. His wife had motor seizures and so Professor Jackson had plenty of opportunity to study them. The seizures often start in the face region of the cortex and then the abnormal activity spreads out along the motor area progressively involving different areas of the body. It spreads from the face area to the thumb and hand and then through the arm down into the rest of the body. This spread is often called a 'march'. Some people may have weakness in the affected limb after a motor seizure for a number of hours, or even occasionally days. This weakness is called a Todd's paralysis, after the Dr Todd whose statue can be seen in the forecourt of Kings College Hospital in South London.

A partial seizure which arises in the sensory cortex (the part of the brain concerned with sensation) will produce an aura which may be a definite feeling such as itching or tingling, or some sensation that is quite indescribable, though instantly recognizable to you. Auras that take the form of simple flashes or speckles of light arise in the occipital cortex.

Sometimes a partial seizure is minor and very brief, and consists only of the aura. On other occasions, if the seizure spreads further throughout the brain, it may cause longer and more disturbance, perhaps being followed by transient weakness of a limb (Todd's paralysis, see above) or a temporary inability to find words (dysphasia). But usually there is no loss of consciousness during the seizure.

Complex Partial Seizures

Complex partial seizures, like simple partial seizures, always begin with an aura but, unlike simple partial seizures, they always produce some disturbance of consciousness. Many complex partial seizures originate in the temporal lobe of the brain, the part of the brain that is involved in emotions, feelings and memory.

Seizures that start in the temporal lobe often begin with a feeling arising in the stomach and moving up to the throat, called an epigastric aura. This is usually accompanied by a sensation of fear which can be so intense that the person fears they are going to die. Less often there may be an aura of taste or smell, usually unpleasant, or of some simple sound such as hummings or clicks. There may be feelings of *déjà vu*, that is, an intense feeling of recognition or a feeling that you know what is going to happen. Some people describe it as a feeling of reincarnation. There may even be a sensation that the world is quite unrecognizable (*jamais vu*). Memories may be triggered off as part of the aura and, very rarely, intensely pleasant mystical, or even sexual feelings can arise.

Sometimes the seizure does not spread, so that it consists only of the aura, and a few people have complex partial seizures which are *always* limited to an aura. But usually the seizure spreads out from its focus through the brain. As it spreads the person starts to behave oddly, and quite automatically. They are unaware of what is happening to them or what they are doing. To begin with they will perform simple pieces of behaviour, like lipsmacking or turning around in circles. After a few seconds the activity has spread further in the brain and the person may perform more complex actions, such as standing up or sitting down or walking about, but they will still be performing automatically. Gradually these actions become even more complex and often quite bizarre, but they show that the person is starting to respond to the environment around them. They may open doors, go outside, and even cross roads. Slowly this behaviour merges into normal behaviour and consciousness gradually returns.

Sometimes a partial seizure may spread so rapidly through a wide area of the brain that it becomes generalized and there is a tonic clonic convulsion. This is called a secondarily generalized seizure.

People who have simple partial or complex partial seizures have one great advantage over those with generalized tonic clonic (*grand mal*) seizures; because of the warning aura they know that a seizure is beginning. So they have time to manoeuvre themselves out of danger – maybe sit down somewhere safe, or put down anything hot or breakable that they are carrying. Many people even manage to develop various techniques to abort their seizures at this stage so that they do not spread any further, and there is no loss of consciousness (see pp.93–110)

Who has epilepsy?

At least one person in 200 (about 300,000 in the UK) suffers from epilepsy, and this is probably a conservative estimate. The figure may be nearly as high as one person in 100.

Epilepsy is very much a disease of the young, partly because the brain is always more excitable in children than it is in adults. If you are going to develop epilepsy, you are most likely to do so in childhood or adolescence. About one quarter of people with epilepsy will have developed the condition by the time they start primary school at the age of five; half will have done so by the time they move on to secondary school at 11. By the age of 18, three-quarters of those who are going to develop the condition will have done so, and, by the age of 20,

90 per cent. There is a further and final peak in middle to old age, this time because of damage to the brain by degenerative disease.

EPILEPSY AND INHERITANCE

Epilepsy runs in families, but inheritance is not the only or even the most important factor involved in the development of seizures. A few types of epilepsy are directly inherited. These inherited epilepsies, of which the most common is tuberous sclerosis (Bourneville's disease), are often accompanied by mental retardation. However, they form only a tiny proportion (about 1 per cent) of all cases of epilepsy. More commonly what you inherit is not epilepsy itself, but a *tendency* to have seizures because your brain is more excitable than normal. So if you have a close relative who suffers from the condition, your own chances of developing epilepsy are slightly higher than average. If you have one parent with the disease your chances of developing it yourself increase to one in 40. And if both parents are affected, the chances are greater still – about one in 20, though this statistic does vary with the type of epilepsy you have.

The genes which determine brain excitability, and which are inherited, have their strongest effect in childhood. That is why most people who develop epilepsy do so then. Excitability 'peaks' at the age of about 16, and thereafter the brain becomes progressively less excitable. This kind of inherited epilepsy used to be called 'idiopathic epilepsy', meaning simply that no one knew what caused it.

Other developmental changes are now thought to be important causes of epilepsy. During the second three months of pregnancy, as the brain develops, cells migrate from one position in the brain to another. Sometimes this migration goes wrong and leads to a condition known as heterotopia. In some people these areas of heterotopia are intensely epileptogenic (that is, very likely to give rise to seizures). Another common congenital (developmental) cause of epilepsy is the dysembryoplastic neuroepithelial tumour, or DNT, a lesion which is found most frequently in the temporal lobe though it can occur elsewhere in the brain.

Common causes of epilepsy

Even if you have inherited a tendency to seizures, you will not necessarily develop epilepsy. Nearly always there has to be some other 'insult' to the brain, usually in the form of damage through head injury or an infection such as encephalitis or lack of oxygen. This kind of damage to the brain can leave a small 'scar', which later acts as a focus for seizures – an area from which seizures can arise. Where the damage is makes a difference to your chances of developing epilepsy: an injury to the frontal and temporal lobes is more likely to cause seizures than damage to the occipital and parietal lobes at the back of the brain.

Childhood epilepsy
When epilepsy develops in infancy or very early in childhood, it is often because there has been some damage to the brain during pregnancy or birth. The damage is usually caused because the baby has been deprived of oxygen, most frequently during the pregnancy, but sometimes during the delivery of the baby. More rarely, damage is due to some developmental defect in the brain.

Seizures due to head injury
Head injury can lead to epilepsy at any age, and is one of the most common causes in young adults. There is usually some loss of memory immediately after a head injury (called post-traumatic amnesia), and one way of measuring the severity of a head injury is by the length of this post-traumatic amnesia. About five per cent of people who have a head injury severe enough to cause loss of memory for half an hour after the injury

eventually develop epilepsy. More than half of these have their first fit within one year of the injury, and three-quarters within three years. Seizures can make their first appearance even later than this. If the injury has penetrated the skull the chances of epilepsy developing are much greater.

Epilepsy is less likely to develop, however, when seizures occur soon after the injury (within a week). These early seizures are much less likely to recur, and much more likely to be simple partial seizures, often limited to a twitching in the hand or face.

Seizures due to febrile convulsions
A few people develop complex partial seizures, usually in childhood and less frequently in adolescence, as a result of febrile convulsions in childhood. Febrile convulsions (see p.155) run in families: they are *grand mal* convulsions which sometimes occur in a few young children when they are running a high temperature. They are nearly always harmless, and most children outgrow them by the time they are three or four years old. But a few children who have very severe or prolonged febrile convulsions do develop epilepsy later in life. This is because during prolonged convulsions the brain may have been temporarily starved of oxygen when the child had difficulty in breathing during a seizure. Such oxygen deprivation can cause brain damage, nearly always in the temporal lobe, which is the part of the brain most easily injured by lack of oxygen. There is some debate as to whether this damage is due entirely to the shortage of oxygen, or whether it actually occurs because there is already some developmental abnormality present in this part of the brain beforehand. In either case the outcome is the same: after a prolonged febrile convulsion this area of the brain is damaged, and from this damage complex partial seizures later arise.

Seizures in adulthood
The biggest worry of anyone who has a first seizure in adulthood is that it is due to a brain tumour. It is true that a fit is often the first sign of a brain tumour. But a brain tumour is still a very rare

cause of seizures in adults. Even in the 50–55 age group, when brain tumours are most common, about 85 per cent of cases of epilepsy will have some other cause – such as cerebro-vascular disease. Epilepsy may be caused by the blockage of a small blood vessel within the brain for example, or a small stroke which has left an area of damage. About 80 per cent of cases in which the fits start after the age of 25 can be successfully controlled by drugs.

What triggers off a seizure?
Some things are especially likely to trigger off a seizure. Drowsiness, low blood sugar, even boredom may do it for example. So too may sleep (some people have convulsions only when they are asleep). But many people who have epilepsy discover that a convulsion is often sparked off by some specific and trivial trigger. It may be a particular movement, something they see or hear, or even a mental image or thought or feeling. Once you have discovered what it is that is most likely to trigger off your own seizures you will probably be able to avoid these triggers much of the time and so cut down your seizure frequency. (See pp.93–110.)

What is it like to have a seizure?

'I can't describe my fits since I can't remember them! Some people have a warning before an attack, but my only warning is that I go very vague, which is no help at all, since if you are vague then you do not realize it! The worst bit about having a fit is when you come round: I take ages to regain full consciousness, and it would be marvellous to have someone saying, "You have had a fit, therefore you are lying on the kitchen floor at Mrs Spinks' house." Most people when pressed

will admit that I have had a fit (I usually have to ask the question) but they fail to tell me where I am. Since I am in such a confused state I need all the information I can get at this stage, together with loads of reassurance. ("I am here, I am not going away, you are going to be all right.")'

From Epilepsy 78, British Epilepsy Association – see appendix)

Many people who have epilepsy cannot actually tell you what they feel like during an attack, because they are either unconscious or confused during it, and have little or no memory of it afterwards. If they want to know what actually happens to them during the seizure itself they are dependent on what they are told by other people who have seen them have a seizure. And this is often a real worry.

'I used to worry dreadfully about people seeing me having a seizure. I thought I must look awful, I didn't want anyone to see me like that. Then my doctor suggested to my parents that they take a video of me during an attack so that I could see what actually happened. I really didn't want them to, and when they'd done it I refused to look at it for ages. But in the end I did and it wasn't nearly as bad as I'd expected. I'm not sure quite what I'd imagined but really it was no big deal. After that I didn't worry nearly so much about having a seizure in public.'

WARNINGS AND AURAS

Sometimes seizures occur out of the blue. But many people who have epilepsy have a time before a seizure during which they may feel restless, irritable, depressed or uncomfortable. A few people feel more energetic than usual before a seizure, and have a feeling of well-being.

These feelings or altered behaviour are called the 'prodrome', and they usually build up slowly for hours or even days before the actual fit begins. Prodromes are more common in children than in adults, and are especially common in people who have temporal lobe epilepsy.

The prodrome is quite different from the aura. The prodrome is a warning that a seizure is going to happen sometime in the future: maybe in a few hours, maybe in as much as three days. But the aura means that the seizure has actually begun. The aura is part of the seizure, caused by seizure activity beginning in the brain. Anyone who has epilepsy may discover that they usually have a prodromal, warning phase, but you will only have an aura if you have simple partial or complex partial seizures – auras do not occur as part of a generalized or *grand mal* seizure.

Even if the person about to have the seizure does not realize that they are in any way different during their prodrome, the people around them may notice some change in their mood or behaviour. Mothers of children who have epilepsy often say that they can tell when their child is going to have a fit. One mother told me:

> *'I can always tell when Mick's going to have a fit, though I honestly can't tell you just how I know. A day or so before I may feel there's something about the way he's looking at me. His eyes seem different. Or he just behaves "differently" somehow, perhaps seems a bit duller than usual, though I doubt if anyone else but me or his dad would notice it.'*

AFTER THE SEIZURE

Most people feel tired or confused for a while after a seizure, and after a tonic clonic or complex partial seizure they may remember little of what has happened. Even if you have no memory of your seizure, there may be one or two painful reminders. Aches and pains in the muscles are common after a tonic clonic seizure because of the muscle spasms that go on during the seizure. Sometimes people pass urine during a seizure. Your tongue or cheek may be sore if it was bitten during the seizure and there may be blood around your mouth. However, even if you fall and hurt yourself you may notice that the injury does not hurt when you recover consciousness, and may not do so for anything up to an hour. This is because during a major convulsion the body releases its own naturally-produced pain-relieving substances, endorphins. People seldom injure themselves during a partial complex seizure unless they were holding a boiling kettle or hot drink at the time the seizure started, or walk into danger during an epileptic automatism (see below).

Consciousness is recovered slowly after a tonic clonic seizure, leaving you feeling confused, disturbed, sleepy and frequently with a headache. Probably you will want to sleep, and will wake up after about two hours, usually feeling better. Although most people feel back to normal the next day, for some the after-effects last longer, and a few people say they do not feel right for a week or more.

Some people find there is a temporary change in their behaviour – for example the way they speak or how they feel – after a seizure. What this is will depend on where the seizure starts. It might be a mood change: a patient of mine used to feel depressed after a seizure, and it was sometimes four or five days before her mood returned to normal. If your seizures start in the speech area of your brain, then this area will be disturbed for a while after the seizure. People who have this kind of speech disturbance say that for an hour or so after a seizure, though they know what they want to say, what comes out is gobbledegook. The feelings most people report are of tiredness and confusion.

EPILEPTIC AUTOMATISMS

Daniel's mother saw him off to school as usual one morning. He took his normal route, dawdling and stopping, as he usually did, to look at the mountain bike he hoped to get for his birthday in the showroom window, so that he was overtaken, by his form master.

'Morning, Daniel. Are we going to see you on time this morning, do you think?'

'I expect so, Mr Phelps. I'll be along in a moment.'

But Daniel wasn't along in a moment. When, by assembly time, he still hadn't turned up, Mr Phelps was worried. After assembly he went to the headmaster, who phoned first Daniel's parents, and then, when it was discovered that he hadn't gone back home, the police.

In fact it was Daniel's father, driving desperately around the town searching for his son, who spotted him some three quarters of an hour later. He was standing on a bridge, looking down into a river.

'Daniel! What happened to you? Where've you been?'

Daniel looked bemused.

'What time is it, Dad? Oh gosh, not 10 o'clock. I'll be late for school again.'

Daniel remembered talking to Mr Phelps. But after that he had no memory of what had happened to him until he found himself looking down into the river. During that time he had walked about two miles and crossed several quite busy roads.

Daniel's is a fairly unusual case of epileptic automatism after a complex partial seizure, but it is not *that* unusual. There are numerous examples of people performing complex acts in a state of confusion, during or immediately after a seizure, usually a generalized or complex partial seizure. Most of these automatisms are brief, lasting only a few seconds. They seldom last longer than a few minutes but can, rarely, continue for as much as an hour.

If someone had stopped Daniel and spoken to him while he was wandering through the town they would have noticed that he seemed out of touch with his surroundings, and looked dazed or vacant. Daniel would probably not have responded if he had been spoken to, or he might have given some incoherent or irrational reply.

However, an epileptic automatism is usually less dramatic than Daniel's experience. The person is more likely to perform simple, repetitive, rather clumsy movements. They may pull at their clothes, repeatedly rub their face or fiddle with something. Sometimes they may perform more complex actions, such as walking about the room, searching for something in a drawer, dressing or undressing. But only occasionally is an automatism, like Daniel's, so seemingly purposeful and co-ordinated that it is difficult to believe that it has been carried out entirely automatically, in a state of such deep confusion that the person does not realize what they are doing and afterwards has no memory at all of what they have done. My own favourite account of an automatism concerns an organist who had an attack while playing the organ in church for a carol concert. He suddenly stopped playing, gave the con-gregation three minutes of uninterrupted jazz, and then, the seizure over, continued with the carol he had been playing as though nothing had happened.

STATUS EPILEPTICUS

Status epilepticus is a prolonged seizure or continuous series of seizures. It is a medical emergency. Not everybody who has epilepsy will suffer from *status epilepticus*. It usually occurs in people who have frontal lobe epilepsy. It is rare for such seizures to arise from other parts of the brain, but because it is so dangerous anyone who has close contact with someone who has epilepsy must be able to recognize it and know what to do.

Normally when someone has a seizure, the brain responds by becoming less excitable for a while, so that another seizure is less likely. However seizures sometimes occur one after the other with only a small gap between them. Like *status epilepticus* these so-called 'serial seizures' may also require urgent medical help, but if the person having the seizures has time to recover between them, the situation does not have quite the degree of urgency of someone who is in *status epilepticus*.

If, on the other hand, the seizures follow hard on one another, occurring so often that the person has no time to recover from one before the next one begins, then it is important to get help as quickly as possible. In true *status epilepticus* the seizures become continuous, so there is no gap between them and the person remains unconscious, convulsing all the while. They may be unable to breathe properly, and the lack of oxygen may lead to brain damage. It is essential to seek help immediately. (For *Emergency Aid* see pp.132–5).

Myths about epilepsy

Epilepsy is a psychiatric disorder or mental illness

It used to be thought that epilepsy was linked to the phases of the moon (hence the origin of the word 'lunatic'). The truth is that epilepsy is a medical condition with a physical cause. People with uncomplicated epilepsy are no more likely to suffer psychiatric disorders than anyone else.

You can tell someone with epilepsy because they have a typical epileptic personality

In the middle of the last century when little was known about epilepsy it was thought that epilepsy was always inherited and always led to a deterioration of the brain and to imbecility and crime. At that time there was no treatment for epilepsy and it was very common for people with severe epilepsy to fall and suffer head injury during their seizures. Many became brain damaged because of these frequent injuries. Later, at the turn of the century, the only anticonvulsant which was available was bromide. At that time it was not possible to monitor the amount of bromide in the blood and so people had very high bromide levels and became toxic, with a consequent deterioration in their behaviour and intelligence. It was these two factors which led to the myth that all epileptics had the same deteriorating personality. We now know that unless there is associated brain damage, people with epilepsy have personalities which are like anybody else.

All patients with epilepsy are violent or criminals

This myth is really an extension of the previous one. At the turn of the century some people became violent either because they were suffering from bromide poisoning, or because they had become brain damaged by frequent falls during severe, uncontrolled seizures.

The myth was perpetuated for a time because some early studies of people in prison found that there were more people with epilepsy than would be expected. However, it is now thought that, in many cases, the epilepsy was caused because of head injuries. It was also demonstrated that their personality was such that even before they had epilepsy, they tended to get into fights. Taking this into account, the number of people with epilepsy who are in prison is no greater than in the general population. The truth is that people with epilepsy are no more likely to be violent or criminal than the rest of the population.

People who have epilepsy are mentally handicapped

This is untrue. Although many people who have learning difficulties also have epilepsy, only a few people who have epilepsy also have learning difficulties. These are the few who have severe brain damage, which causes both their learning difficulties and their seizures. But few people with epilepsy have brain damage of this severity.

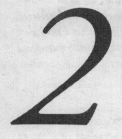

chapter two

Diagnosing Epilepsy

'*I had my first fit at the age of 12. I was on board ship at the time with the Girl Guides. Since it was my first trip abroad, and there was a force eight gale raging in the North Sea, no one thought that it was anything more than a childish convulsion. No one told me about it either. I had this incredible dream of lying in a cabin wearing a friend's blazer. No one said, 'That's not a dream, that happened to you yesterday.' Why there was all this secrecy I never knew.*

'*I returned home from my trip abroad, and proceeded to relate all to my parents. "You haven't told me everything," said my mother. "You didn't tell me you were ill while you were away." No one was more astonished than me. Despite my protests I was led off to see the doctor, who gave me tablets to take, told me never to forget them, and said no more.*

'*A year later I went off to camp with the Guides again. I remember being sent to the farmhouse to collect eggs and bread, with another girl to help carry. "Thank goodness Sarah had the eggs," was the comment of the day, since I had a fit just outside the farmhouse door. My mother was sent for and suggestions were made that perhaps it was being away from home that "upset" me. To her everlasting credit my mother asked me what I felt about the whole matter, and I was allowed to stay at the camp. It was bad enough being the "different" girl who had the fit: I didn't want to be the "different girl who went home" too.*

'I had my third fit a few months after that and went to see a specialist at a London hospital. "Epilepsy," he confirmed after tests had been done. It was almost a relief to know that I had a recognizable condition, and was not just having "funny turns" every so often . . .'

(From Epilepsy '78, British Epilepsy Association – see appendix)

Plenty of people will recognize and empathize with this feeling of relief when a vague feeling of being under the weather or a series of odd or inexplicable symptoms turns out to have a solid basis in medical fact. Whatever the diagnosis, once you know what is wrong you can start to face it and deal with it.

However, a diagnosis of epilepsy is not one to be made lightly. Once it is made, the person concerned is given a 'label' that may affect their chances of employment or lose them various privileges – a driving licence for example. It means, too, that they will have to start a regime of drug-taking that may continue for months or even years.

Another problem is that epilepsy is not a simple disease and it is not always easy to diagnose. There is no such thing as a 'typical' case of epilepsy. It can take many forms and have many different symptoms; there is no one simple test for it. This is one reason (among several) why people who have epilepsy dislike being lumped together and referred to as 'epileptics'. It is a meaningless label as well as an insulting one.

What to do for a first fit

The first time you or anyone in your family has a fit, you should consult a doctor. Often there may have been some obvious reason for the fit (if it followed alcohol withdrawal after a period of heavy drinking, for example, or if it occurred in a child during a high fever), and in this case your doctor may not suggest any further investigations or recommend any anticonvulsant medication. However, if there was no obvious reason for the fit, or if the doctor feels it is necessary, he or she will almost certainly suggest that you undergo a thorough investigation to discover whether your fits are likely to recur and whether there is any underlying cause for them that can be treated.

MAKING THE DIAGNOSIS

The diagnosis of epilepsy is made by looking at what happens during the seizures. There are plenty of other reasons besides epilepsy for sudden attacks of unconsciousness or odd behaviour, and all of these will have to be ruled out before a final diagnosis of epilepsy can be made. Fainting, breath-holding attacks, night terrors, migraine, episodes of day-dreaming or inattentiveness in schoolchildren, aggressive outbursts in disturbed adolescents – all of these can be, and quite often are, mistaken for epilepsy.

So before making the diagnosis your doctor will want to have as much information as possible about you. You'll be asked whether anyone else in your family has ever suffered from epilepsy. You will be given a full physical examination, and your doctor will want to know your medical history and exactly what happened when you had your attack. Your own recollection of events and eyewitness accounts of anyone who was with you at the time will all help the doctor decide whether what you experienced was, in fact, an epileptic attack, and if so, what kind. These are some of the questions you will probably be asked:

- **What was happening at the time of the seizure?**
  Were you particularly tired, for example? Had you been drinking or had you missed a meal and were very hungry? Were you watching television, or were you at a disco? Was it very hot? Did it happen after you had just stood up and were feeling faint?

- **Have you recently had a blow on the head?**
  Or have you at any time in the past suffered a head injury severe enough to render you unconscious or keep you in hospital for observation? Any significant head injury may increase the chances of you developing epilepsy in the future.
- **Does any member of your family suffer from epilepsy?**
- **Do you suffer from any chronic illness?**
- **Have you recently had an infectious illness?**
- **Have you been under particular pressure lately, or been very worried about anything?**
- **What did you or those around you notice about the seizure itself?**
  What was the very first thing you noticed when the seizure started? Was it an odd smell or taste, for example, some weird sensation or thought or an involuntary movement like the twitching of a hand or arm? If there was any jerking or twitching, how did it spread? What part of the body was affected before you lost consciousness? Did it affect one side or both sides of your body and how long did it last? Be as specific as you can. It is these observations which will help your doctor decide which part of your brain gave rise to the seizure.
- **Did you fall to the ground during the seizure?**
- **Did you lose consciousness during the seizure?**
- **What happened immediately after the seizure?**
  If anyone was with you, did they notice whether you changed colour? Did you seem confused after the seizure and if so, for how long? As you were coming round, did they notice any difficulties in your speech? Was it slurred, for example, or did you have difficulty finding the right words?
- **How did you feel after the attack?**
  Did you notice any weakness in your limbs after the attack? Did you have a headache or feel depressed? Did you fall asleep after the attack? Or did you feel much better afterwards?
- **How much memory do you have of the event?**

Referral to a specialist

Once it has been decided that what happened to you was, in all probability, a seizure, your doctor will want to discover whether it was due to some underlying cause that should be treated, and whether the fits are likely to recur.

It is possible that if this is your first fit the doctor may adopt a 'wait and see' policy. But they may – and certainly if you have had one or more previous attacks, they will – refer you to a neurologist.

Doctors, like gardeners, have their own fields of expertise. Medicine moves so fast nowadays that it is virtually impossible for a GP to be up to date with every new development in every field of medicine. Unless your GP has a special interest in epilepsy it is quite possible that their ideas about treating the condition may not be right up at the frontier of current thinking. Your GP may, for example, want to start treating you without referring you for further investigations. It is not unheard of for a GP to say to a patient, 'You've got epilepsy. Go away and keep taking these tablets.'

This used to be normal practice because it used to be thought that the cause of epilepsy was unimportant. Indeed, in most cases it was believed that there was no cause to be found, and that most instances of epilepsy were 'idiopathic', that is, that there was no known cause for them. Investigations were pointless because so far as treatment was concerned the end result was much the same: 'Keep on taking the tablets.'

Things are rather different now. New methods of imaging the brain have been developed which can produce a highly detailed picture of our most complex organ. The use of these new methods has shown one thing very clearly, and that is that epilepsy usually occurs for some reason. The old concept of idiopathic epilepsy, epilepsy without a cause, no longer holds true.

A neurologist will carry out tests to detect abnormalities either in the structure of your brain or in the way it is working. You will also be given blood tests, which can indicate whether there is any medical reason which might account for your seizure. These routine tests are all quite straightforward and painless and carry no risk. Usually the tests will give detailed information about the cause of the epilepsy.

Discovering the cause of your epilepsy is important for two reasons. To begin with, it may affect the choice of treatment. Until you are certain what is causing the epilepsy it is not possible to choose the appropriate treatment. And secondly, it helps most people who have epilepsy to know *why* it developed. It helps their families too. Whenever a child is ill, for example, parents tend to blame themselves, however illogical this may be. They want to know how it happened, and to be able to explain it to themselves.

Whether or not you are referred to a neurologist may also depend on whether or not you ask for a referral. Some people feel easier if they have as much information as possible about what is wrong with them; others are happy simply to accept what they are told and to leave all decisions up to their doctor. Neither approach is either right or wrong; it is very much a matter of your own particular personality. However, if you ask to be referred to a neurologist who has a special interest in epilepsy and your doctor seems reluctant to do so, it is reasonable to ask why. If they continually refuse to refer you, it might be worth changing your doctor to one who has a broader understanding of epilepsy.

Special investigations

Once you have been referred to a specialist, what kind of investigations will you have to undergo? The first and most important test you will be given is electroencephalography. This may be enough to confirm the diagnosis of epilepsy and suggest what treatment you should be given. If more information is needed you may be given a CT scan and possibly an MRI scan, though the latter is not available everywhere. And in a few specialized units you may be given psychometric testing – tests of intelligence and memory to see whether any particular area of the brain is functioning less well than the others.

ELECTROENCEPHALOGRAM

An electroencephalogram (EEG) records the electrical activity of the brain; your 'brain waves'. Abnormalities of electrical activity show up on the EEG recording in about 75 per cent of people who have epilepsy. But an abnormal EEG does not necessarily mean that you have epilepsy, and neither does a normal EEG prove that you do *not* have epilepsy.

An EEG recording takes about one hour. Small silver discs (electrodes) will be attached to your scalp with a special glue. This does not involve any shaving of the hair, although your hair may have little tacky bits in it afterwards and need to be washed. During the recording you will be asked to do various things which are likely to provoke epileptic activity, including opening and closing your eyes, overbreathing and sitting in front of a flickering disco-like lamp (a strobe).

Sleep enhances epileptic activity in some people who have perfectly normal EEGs while they are awake. If your sleep EEG is to be recorded, you will probably be asked to take a sleeping tablet (seconal) to help you sleep during the day in the unfamiliar laboratory surroundings.

The specialist's report on your EEG may mention the following terms:

- **Paroxysmal activity**
- **Spike and wave**
  These first two observations are both suggestive of generalized epilepsy.
- **Focal spikes** These indicate that there is abnormal activity in one part of the brain, suggesting partial epilepsy.

31

- **Generalized slow activity** This often indicates that there is some underlying brain dysfunction, though it is not necessarily epilepsy.

EEG TELEMETRY

Sometimes it is important to know exactly which part of the brain is giving rise to seizures, and what type of electrical activity accompanies them. And sometimes, too, it is useful to be able to correlate what is going on in the brain with actual behaviour during a seizure. This can be helpful if it is thought that seizures may have an emotional cause and are not due to epilepsy (see non-epileptic seizures, pp.103–110). This kind of information can only be obtained by watching the changes in behaviour that occur during the seizure as it happens and at the same time recording the electrical activity going on in the brain.

Unfortunately, seizures cannot be created to order. It is only by doing a continuous EEG recording over a long period and videoing the person the whole time that there is a good chance of capturing one or two seizures. This process of continuous seizure monitoring is called telemetry, and is carried out in a special telemetry unit. The telemetry unit is just like an ordinary EEG department but is sited in a hospital ward.

Most units now use cable telemetry, which is felt to be more reliable than radiotelemetry. In cable telemetry the EEG electrodes are fixed to your head just as they are for an ordinary routine EEG recording. The wires from the electrodes are gathered together and lead to a little amplifier which is usually strapped to your chest. From this amplifier a cable leads to a plug in the wall and from here the signals are taken to an EEG machine and tape recorder. The lead is long enough for you to be able to get out of bed and wander around, but you are not encouraged to do too much wandering, as you always have to stay within the field of view of the video camera and it is best if you sit still in a chair as the quality of the recordings is diminished by movement.

Most units will let you unplug the cable from the wall and replug it in the ward day-room so that you can at least have a change of scenery and sit and talk to other patients, though you will still be within range of a video camera. There are also video cameras monitoring the dining area. However, you are able to unplug yourself and have a few unmonitored moments of privacy if you want to have a bath or go to the lavatory. You will usually stay in the telemetry unit for one or two weeks, being recorded 24 hours a day. Obviously, this is a very expensive procedure and so it is not carried out unless there is a very good reason for it.

Another form of telemetry, less popular but still sometimes used, is 24 hour cassette tape monitoring. Electrodes are placed on the head in exactly the same way as in cable telemetry, but the wires lead to a portable tape recorder strapped round your waist, which records your brain activity throughout the 24 hours. You can wear this anywhere, so it allows you to stay at home, or go to work or school.

The disadvantage of this system is that because you are moving around normally all the time the recording is taking place, the quality of the recording is not as good as in cable telemetry. More important, if you have a seizure it will not be captured on video. Instead, you or some observer close to you will have to make an accurate and detailed seizure and activity log – a record of your activity throughout the 24 hours. This can then be correlated with the EEG recording, which has a time clock. It is a tedious and time-consuming process and the results are sometimes difficult to interpret. Inevitably, it does not yield as much information as cable telemetry.

MRI SCAN OR CT SCAN

Both MRI (Magnetic Resonance Imaging) and CT (Compu-terized Tomography) are ways of producing images of the structure of the brain. CT does this by measuring the way X-rays are absorbed by the brain. MRI does it in a more complex way, by surrounding the brain with a strong magnetic field and assessing the way that the water in the brain (which is composed of charged particles called protons) responds to high-frequency pulses of radiomagnetic energy. Sometimes the radiologist will ask for an injection of 'contrast' material to be injected intravenously. This substance will outline the major blood vessels in the brain and will show up any abnormalities in them.

Neither of these procedures is either harmful or uncomfortable, and both give a very good picture of the main structures of the brain. The radiologist who interprets the films will be able to tell whether the fluid-filled cavities in the brain (the ventricles), are normal in size and position, whether the convolutions of the brain are normal in shape and form, and whether or not there is an abnormality in the substance of the brain such as a tumour, a vascular anomaly or a developmental abnormality.

Although all major hospitals now have CT scanners, MRI scans are only available in a few units. However, it is always worth having an MRI scan if you can, because it can give information about the structure of the brain which the CT scan cannot give. Twenty per cent of people who have normal CTs are found to have abnormalities when they are given MRI scans.

In particular, the MRI scan can show the structure of the hippocampus and amygdala, which is an area in the temporal lobe of the brain from which seizures very commonly arise. MRI scanning can also show developmental abnormalities which are difficult to see on the CT. This is a technology which is developing very rapidly. A new technique called MRI spectroscopy shows chemical abnormalities in some cells, indicating the site of the seizure focus.

Having a CT scan

Having a CT scan is rather like having to lie with your head in a huge washing machine. You lie on a bed with your head inside a metal structure which rotates around it, sending out X-rays all the time. Even if you dislike being in confined spaces, you probably will not mind the CT scanner. The machine feels very open and there is plenty of space around you so that you should not feel at all constricted.

The whole scanning process is very quick and should be over within five minutes. However, it will take considerably longer for the computers to build up the brain pictures for the radiologist. While the scan is being taken it is essential that you lie absolutely still as any movement distorts the image.

Because X-rays are dangerous for an unborn child, CT scans are never given to anyone who is pregnant. Women are always asked to fill in a questionnaire before being scanned, letting the radiologist know the date of their last period.

Having an MRI scan

Having an MRI scan is a more complicated procedure. Because very strong magnetic fields, several million times stronger than the earth's magnetic field, are used during MRI scanning, all watches, credit cards and metal materials such as belt buckles have to be left outside the scanning room.

You will have to fill in a questionnaire before having the scan. If you have a heart pacemaker you will not be able to have an MRI scan. You will be asked about the work that you do, too. If your job involves working with metal there is a risk that metal filings may have worked their way into your eyes. In this case, scanning may be dangerous as the magnetic field is strong enough to pull out the filings and damage the eye. Metal clips in the brain from previous intercranial surgery will also stop you having a scan. Metal bridges in the teeth and metal pins in the shoulders or hips will not usually prevent you having a scan, but you must note these on the form.

An MRI scanner looks quite different from a CT scanner. It consists of a long tube into which your whole body slides. It does seem constricting, and makes many people feel claustrophobic. If you tend to feel panicky in confined spaces, it is worth mentioning this to the doctor. You can then be given a sedative half an hour before the scan to make you feel more relaxed.

The MRI scanner also makes a terrible racket – a very loud drumming, thumping noise – while it is working. Most units offer you headphones so that you can play a tape of your choice, so make sure you take one with you. In fact, the noise is often so loud that you cannot hear the tape, but it is nice to know it is playing!

MRI scans take much longer than CT scans. The whole process of filling in the form, emptying your pockets, going into the scanner, being scanned, coming out again and being reunited with your possessions seldom takes less than an hour. As with the CT scan, it is essential that you lie absolutely still during the scan, as any movement degrades the MRI images. You will have to lie still for at least 20 minutes.

There is as yet no evidence that strong magnetic fields are in any way dangerous. However, because this is still a fairly new method, and it is always best to be on the safe side, MRI scans are not given to pregnant women.

PSYCHOMETRIC TESTS

All of us are good at some things and poor at others. Some people are good at remembering people's faces but can never remember their names. Others are good at art, useless at spelling. Most psychological functions come from specific brain areas and if these areas are damaged, then you may lose some particular ability.

Epileptic seizures often arise from a small area of damaged brain. By assessing someone's different mental skills it is often possible to see which part of the brain may have been damaged. This is done by psychometric testing.

Essentially, psychometric testing involves answering a lot of questions which have been designed to test the functioning of different brain areas. In some you will be asked to write down the answers, in others you will have to give a verbal answer or perform some simple task. All these tests have to be given in a very specialized standard way by a trained neuropsychologist who knows not only how to give them but also how to interpret the results. Sometimes an abnormality of brain functioning can be detected in this way even though nothing has shown up in the EEG or CT scan, and more and more epilepsy units now realize the value of having a trained neuropsychologist as a member of their team. If you are to have psychometric testing, it is important to let the psychologist know if you have had a seizure in the day or so before the tests as this may alter the results.

Doing the tests

The psychologist will sit down opposite you at a table in a quiet room so that you can concentrate on the tests. Usually the first set of tests will assess your general level of intelligence, and also show whether both left and right sides of your brain are working equally well. Some of these tests are mainly verbal, and include vocabulary tests, questions which test your understanding of different situations, and arithmetic tests. In right-handed people these test the functioning of the left side of the brain. Others are to do with your perception of space; they may include tests asking you to analyse the meaning of pictures, cancel out symbols, and put blocks into spatial patterns. They test the functioning of the right side of the brain. These two sets of tests will each be scored, to give two IQ scores, a verbal IQ and a performance (spatial) IQ. In most people these two figures are nearly the same. But if one half of the brain is damaged, then there will be a discrepancy between the two scores.

You will then be asked to do other tests to measure special brain functions. Memory, for example, is situated in a special part of the temporal lobe, the hippocampus. Memory for words is on the left side, and memory for pictures on the right. If there is any damage to the hippocampus on either side of the brain, one of your memory scores will probably be lower than the other.

Damage in other regions of the brain can be tested for in the same way. Your ability to recognize faces, for example, is at the back of the right temporal lobe. Verbal fluency tests (measured by counting the number of words beginning with a given letter that you can say in 5 minutes) will test the left frontal region whereas spatial sequencing tests (such as working your way through a maze) will test the right frontal region. You will not have to do every available test; the psychologist will know from the results of your EEG and brain scanning which area of your brain is likely to be damaged, and the questions you will be asked will be to test the functioning of this particular area.

Do not worry if you fail on the tests. In fact, the tests are graded so that they start easy and then become harder as you go through them, so that at some point you are almost bound to fail. This does not matter. They have to be designed so that no one will find the whole test too easy, however clever they are. The aim is not to see whether you pass or fail, but only to find out whether some parts of your brain are working less efficiently than others.

A neuropsychological session will usually take one to two hours and you will find it quite tiring (but usually quite fun as well) as you have to concentrate for all this time. Sometimes it may not be possible to complete all the tests in one session, and in this case you will be asked to come back another day to finish them.

PET SCANNING

PET (Positron Emission Tomography) is a new method of scanning which is helpful in the diagnosis of epilepsy.

The principle of PET scanning is to see which parts of the brain are active, either by measuring the blood flow through different parts of the brain, or by seeing how actively the different areas of the brain are metabolizing a substance, usually sugar.

To do this, an injection of radioactively-labelled glucose or a dose of radioactively-labelled oxygen in water is given. The radioactivity is taken up more readily by the active areas of the brain. As the radioactivity decays, the PET scanner detects the decay products and calculates where the radioactivity has come from within the brain. The scanner then makes a map of the brain showing the active and inactive metabolic areas. It has been found that areas of the brain which have an active epileptic focus are metabolically less active between seizures, as if the brain were trying to stop the spread of epileptic activity. Not surprisingly, during a seizure this area becomes more active than the surrounding brain. PET scanning is therefore able to give some idea of where seizures are arising.

SPECT or SPET (Single Photon Emission Computer Tomography or Single Photon Emission Tomography) is a less accurate scanning method essentially the same as PET but using a different radioactive chemical which is easier to use. This has the advantage that it can be given during a seizure.

Chapter Three

Treating Epilepsy

*'*P*ills — how I hate them! If you have epilepsy your whole life seems to be governed by pills. It's not that I mind the pills themselves, it's just so difficult always to have to remember to take them. You can't even prolong a holiday or decide to stay with friends on the spur of the moment because you might not have enough tablets with you.'*

(From Epilepsy '78 British Epilepsy Association – see appendix)

The modern treatment of epilepsy

On the surface, the treatment of epilepsy seems little more effective than it did 100 years ago when the first anticonvulsant drugs were introduced. At that time about a third of sufferers lost their fits altogether with drug treatment, a third were improved and a third were no better or worse after treatment.

These figures are much the same today, but even so, the treatment of epilepsy is now very different. To begin with, there is a much wider armoury of drugs, and they have far less damaging side-effects. If one does not suit you or does not control your seizures well, another probably will. You and your doctor, maybe with some trial and error, will eventually be able to find the best drug for you.

Secondly, although we are no nearer to finding a 'cure' for the condition, we do understand it much better. We now have a good idea, for example, of the events within the brain that lead to a seizure. This means that drugs are being developed which can target special areas of the brain and so modify these events and reduce the frequency of seizures.

Thirdly, we do not have to rely only on drugs for treatment. Surgery, for example, which used to be thought of only as the last resort of the desperate, is now a safe and successful option for people who have some types of epilepsy. And if drugs do not work and surgery is inappropriate there are also alternative methods of treatment such as biofeedback, which some sufferers have found helpful.

Finally, there is a new and quite different approach to the treatment of epilepsy which involves modifying a person's behaviour as well as (or in some cases even instead of) giving them drugs. We know now that in many cases seizures do not just happen randomly, but that they are closely related to the person's thoughts, actions, and life style. By studying and analysing how they behave, someone who has epilepsy can often manage to modify their behaviour in a way which will help to control their seizures or even avoid them.

Unfortunately, at the moment these self-help 'behavioural' methods are usually only taught in specialist epilepsy centres, so that most people with epilepsy will never have had the chance to try them out. But this do-it-yourself approach to epilepsy is something that almost everyone can learn, and most people will find helpful. If you want to experiment to see how much control you can learn to exercise over your own seizures, pp.93–110 describe the methods you can use.

Drug treatment of epilepsy

Drugs are always the first line of treatment when a diagnosis of epilepsy has been made. Your doctor will suggest that you take anticonvulsant medication to control your seizures. You do not have to accept the offer, but in almost every case such drugs have a beneficial effect on the frequency and severity of seizures.

Unfortunately, all the drugs used to treat epilepsy have some side-effects, and you will have to weigh these against the advantages of improved seizure control. Whatever drug is chosen, your doctor will aim to minimize the side-effects by giving you the smallest dose that will control your seizures effectively.

If you have occasional or very minor seizures you may find it easier to cope with the seizures than with the side-effects of the drugs. But it is worth remembering that you lose certain privileges if you are subject to fits; you cannot hold a driving licence, for example, and your chances of employment may be affected. There are other things to consider too. Seizures tend to beget seizures; the more you have, the more you are likely to have. Unchecked, your epilepsy may get worse. You also need to remember that epilepsy can, very occasionally, be life threatening. A few people each year die in *status epilepticus* (see p.22) or suffer another rare syndrome called 'sudden death in epilepsy'. This is a condition in which, after a *grand mal* seizure, for reasons that are not fully understood, the brain just stops working and the person dies. The sudden death syndrome occurs very rarely and is mainly confined to young men who refuse to accept a diagnosis of epilepsy, or to take the medication prescribed. Often alcohol plays a part too.

These risks are very small, but they do exist. If you have *grand mal* seizures you may be putting your life on the line if you decide not to take drugs to control your seizures.

HOW DRUGS INTERACT

If you have epilepsy it is quite likely that at times you will regularly be taking more than one drug. It may be that you are prescribed two anticonvulsants, or that you are taking a different kind of drug altogether, for example the contraceptive pill, as well as your anticonvulsant.

Anticonvulsants interact with the actions of many other drugs, and even with each other, sometimes potentiating (increasing) their action, sometimes making them less effective. Alcohol, sedative drugs, anticoagulants and oral contraceptives all interact with some anticonvulsant drugs. The pill, for example, is likely to be less effective if you are taking an anticonvulsant. This does not mean that you cannot take the pill, but it does mean that you should take it under medical supervision for a while so that the dose can be adjusted accordingly (see p.190). Always tell any new doctor that you are taking anticonvulsants.

Tolerance develops to a few anticonvulsant drugs. This means that after you have been taking them for some time, their effect grows weaker. If this happens your doctor will suggest that you take a break from that particular drug. However, when a drug is reintroduced after a 'drug holiday' it may never be quite as effective as it was when you first began to take it.

SIDE-EFFECTS OF DRUGS

All drugs will produce side-effects if they are given in too high a dose (these are called toxic side-effects). But most have a few side-effects even when the recommended therapeutic dose is given. Moreover, a few people have an idiosyncratic reaction to a drug; they respond, sometimes even to a very low dose of the drug, in an individual and atypical way that could not have been predicted.

All anticonvulsants will tend to make you drowsy and affect your powers of concentration. In some cases people around you may notice some personality change or alteration in your behaviour. The drugs may cause a loss of sexual interest too. They can cause a wide range of physical symptoms, including dizziness and nausea. They have often been blamed for causing acne, but most do not deserve this reputation. This is a myth which has probably arisen because a large number of epilepsy sufferers are adolescent – and therefore spotty. Surveys of people with epilepsy have shown that they have no more than their normal share of spots.

Most of the drugs listed below are effective to some extent in all types of seizure and most act by altering the excitability of the brain. Your doctor will try to find the one drug which works best for you, but if you have very severe epilepsy you may need a combination of drugs to establish control. Whatever drug you take, it is important to take it regularly, and not to stop taking it suddenly: suddenly discontinuing the drug may cause seizures, or even lead to *status epilepticus*. If you have epilepsy you will be entitled to an exemption certificate so that you do not have to pay prescription charges for your drugs.

'HALF-LIFE'

You may come across a reference to the 'half-life' of the drug you are taking.

You will be prescribed a dose of a particular drug. As it is absorbed, the level of the drug in your blood will peak before it gradually starts to fall. The 'half-life' is the time it takes for the level to fall back to half its peak level. If a drug has a very short half-life you will need to take frequent doses to keep the blood level high enough to be effective. A drug with a long half-life need be taken less often. A few drugs are available as special slow-release preparations which can therefore be taken less often.

First-line drugs

Your doctor will almost certainly prescribe one of these before trying any other medication. Each has some individual side-effects in addition to those already mentioned which are common to all the drugs, but only a small proportion of people develop these individual side-effects. You will see that the drug you take has two or even more names. The first name given here is the drug's chemical name. The name (or names) given in brackets is its trade name – the drug manufacturer's 'own-brand' version of the drug. Sometimes several drug companies produce their own version of a drug. Usually there is no difference between any of these brands, but it is usually best to stick to one version of a drug if you have found that it suits you.

Whatever drug you are given, you will probably be prescribed a small dose to start with, which will gradually be increased if you suffer no side-effects.

CARBAMAZEPINE (TEGRETOL)

Carbamazepine is one of the best-known and most widely-used anticonvulsants. Most doctors believe that it has the fewest side-effects, and it is thought to be the safest drug for women who are pregnant. So it is the drug your doctor is most likely to try first.

Its main uses are in complex partial seizures and generalized tonic clonic (*grand mal*) seizures, during pregnancy and in people who are depressed, as it tends to brighten mood.

Probably the best preparation to take is Tegretol Retard – this is a slow-release form of the drug, which means you may need only one dose during each 24 hours, at night.

Possible side-effects
- **Rash** If you develop a rash, your doctor will probably keep you on a low dose of the drug for a while and the

chances are that the rash will disappear. A very few people develop a rash so severe that the drug has to be stopped.

- **A low white blood cell count** These cells are the ones which fight infection, and so a low white cell count means that you may be more likely to develop infections. If your white cell count continues to drop your doctor will lower the dose, and some doctors prefer to take patients off the drug. However, my own view is that it is not necessary to withdraw the drug altogether unless the white count does not rise when the dose of the drug is reduced.

- **Water retention, sometimes with swollen ankles and puffy face** This happens because carbamazepine affects the hormone which controls water excretion by the kidneys. This can result in a low – sometimes a very low – blood sodium level. In your three or six-monthly check up your doctor should always measure your blood sodium level. Usually even if you have a very low sodium level it will come back towards normal if the dose of carbamazepine is slightly reduced. However, occasionally this does not occur and then the drug has to be discontinued.

- **Blocks the action of the thyroid gland** Your thyroid may be tested from time to time to check that this is not happening.

- **Reduces the action of other drugs** This is because carbamazepine causes the liver (which is the organ responsible for breaking down most other drugs) to produce more enzymes and so become more active. If you take the contraceptive pill, for example, it will be broken down more rapidly, and in order for it to be effective you will need to take a higher dose.

Toxic side-effects
(These indicate that the dose you are taking is too high.)
Poor balance, double vision and tiredness.

When to avoid
Carbamazepine should not be taken if you have any liver damage, or have responded badly to the drug in the past. Carbamazepine may also be unsuitable if you have some form of heart disease.

PHENYTOIN (EPANUTIN)

Phenytoin is a good anticonvulsant, but is a drug which is unpopular at the moment because of its unpleasant side-effects. It is used to control *grand mal* seizures, and complex partial seizures.

Phenytoin is a drug which is difficult to make up properly. Epanutin is the product of the drug company which was the first to produce this drug. Others have copied them, but not always so successfully. Not long ago, for example, the Australian government decided to save money and recommended the use of cheaper brands of phenytoin. Unfortunately, these different products had different absorption rates, and in consequence many people developed severe seizures. The government finally had to allow the prescription of Epanutin again.

So although there are other, cheaper brands of phenytoin on the market, I would always advise that you stick to Epanutin and make sure that your doctor prescribes it by name.

Possible side-effects
- Rashes
- Slows you down
- Drowsiness
- Roughens facial features
- Swollen gums
- Excessive hairiness
- Tingling in fingers and toes (Peripheral neuritis)
- Leaches calcium from bones
- In high doses, reduces action of other drugs Like Carbamazepine, phenytoin makes the liver more active and produce more enzymes. The contraceptive pill, for

example, may be less effective because it is destroyed more rapidly. In this instance you would have to take a stronger dose of the pill to get the full contraceptive effect (see pp.190–1).

Toxic side-effects
(These indicate that the dose you are taking is too high.) Rapid, jerky eye movements (nystagmus), disturbed balance, tremor. Most importantly, if too high a dose is given, phenytoin stops acting as an anticonvulsant and can actually *induce* seizures.

Double or blurred vision and headaches sometimes occur and, rarely, phenytoin can cause severe confusion and the inability to think clearly. But these side-effects *are* rare, and usually only happen in someone who has taken the drug for a very long time. If they do occur, see your doctor who will probably withdraw the drug.

When to avoid
Phenytoin should be avoided if you are pregnant, and not taken if you have any liver damage or suffer from osteoporosis (weakness of the bones).

SODIUM VALPROATE (EPILIM)

This is a useful drug for controlling generalized seizures (both *grand mal,* and absence seizures) and myoclonic jerks. It is also the drug most often given to prevent febrile convulsions in susceptible children. Sodium valproate has a short half-life (see p.44), so it may need to be taken three times a day to be effective. However, you will probably be given the 'Epilim Chrono' form. This is a slow-release preparation which you will probably only need to take once a day (although some patients like to take it twice a day). It is so much more convenient that I no longer prescribe ordinary valproate any more.

Sodium valproate interacts with another commonly prescribed drug, lamotrigine (see p.51), preventing its breakdown. In effect, this means that too much lamotrigine will accumulate in the blood. So if you are taking both drugs your doctor will want to check your serum level of lamotrigine regularly to make sure it is not too high.

Possible side-effects

- **Hair loss** If you take sodium valproate it is worth looking at your comb after you have combed your hair to see if you seem to be losing more hair than usual. Hair loss is sometimes dose-dependent; as sodium valproate is a good drug, it is usually worth trying a lower dosage before stopping the drug completely. If you do continue with the drug, the hair loss may become so bad that you will need to wear a wig, and when finally you do stop the drug and your hair grows back, it is likely to be of a different colour and finer texture.

- **Change in colour and texture of hair** This is usually associated with hair loss, although it can occur on its own. Again a reduction of drug dosage may help.

- **Tremor** This is a difficult side-effect to treat as it is seldom dose-dependent (although it can be a toxic symptom, due to too high a dose). I have found that if tremor occurs then it is best to withdraw the drug rather than to persevere with lower dosages.

- **Weight gain** This is one of the most difficult side-effects to deal with. Most people are upset when they put on too much weight, and weight gain is particularly distressing for adolescents, who are, even in the best of circumstances, very self-conscious about the way they look. Unfortunately sodium valproate is usually very effective in this age group and very widely used. In my experience, weight gain cannot be avoided simply by reducing the dose of the drug. If it is very troublesome a change of drug is the only satisfactory solution.

Toxic side-effects

(These indicate that the dose you are taking is too high.)
Poor balance, double vision, tiredness and tremor. Very
occasionally, sodium valproate can have a serious effect on
blood clotting. Children given the drug will be watched
carefully as, rarely, it can cause liver damage in a very
special group of young children.

When to avoid

Sodium valproate should be avoided if possible during pregnancy, or if you have ever had liver damage. It should be taken
with care with phenobarbitone or primidone, as the combination can make you very drowsy. If you do become pregnant
while taking sodium valproate, you should certainly discuss this
with your doctor (see p.195).

ETHOSUXIMIDE (ZARONTIN)

Ethosuximide is an alternative to sodium valproate as the drug of
first choice to control absence seizures (*petit mal*). Both drugs
are probably equally effective, but sodium valproate has the
advantage that it controls generalized seizures too, so if you suffer
both types of seizure, sodium valproate is probably the drug you
will be given.

Possible side-effects

These are few. The most likely are:

- Nausea
- Dizziness
- Headache
- Drowsiness

Very rarely adults may also experience hallucinations (seeing
things or hearing voices when no one is there) or suffer
depression.

When to avoid
Ethosuximide should not be used during pregnancy, if you are breast-feeding or if you have ever had liver or kidney damage.

Second-line drugs

LAMOTRIGINE (LAMICTAL)

Lamotrigine is a fairly new drug, and is used for both partial complex seizures and generalized seizures. Its side-effects are generally mild. Its main advantage over other anti-convulsants is that it does not produce the same 'slowing-down' effect on thinking (though a few people do find that high doses of the drug have a sedative effect). In fact, for most people it is an alerting drug – some say it makes them feel as if they have had ten cups of coffee. However, if the dose is reduced a little, this feeling usually passes off. Some people have reported that lamotrigine increases sexual interest. This would be good news, but so far trials of the drug have not confirmed it.

Many people develop a rash when they first start to take lamotrigine, and the drug has to be withdrawn. This is a pity because it is a good drug, and the problem can usually be avoided if the drug is given in a low dose (25mg) for at least the first two weeks. If your doctor starts you on a higher dose it would be worth drawing this fact to his attention.

Possible side-effects
- Rash
- Hyper-alertness

Toxic side-effects
(These indicate that the dose you are taking is too high.) Poor balance, double vision, tremor and, in high doses, tiredness.

51

BENZODIAZEPINES

The benzodiazepines – Diazepam (Valium), Clobazam (Frisium) and Clomazepam (Rivotril) – are a group of drugs which reduce the excitability of the brain by mimicking the effect of the inhibitory brain chemical GABA (see p.55).

DIAZEPAM (VALIUM)

Diazepam is a benzodiazepine whose main use is to terminate *status epilepticus* or febrile convulsions. It is usually given intravenously, either by your doctor or in a hospital casualty department. The main disadvantage of intravenous diazepam is that it can suppress your ability to breathe. If this happens you will have to be taken to the intensive-care unit and your breathing watched and if necessary regulated by the use of a ventilator. Although such a side-effect is unlikely, it happens sufficiently often for doctors to be very aware of the possibility.

A safer way of giving diazepam as an emergency treatment for people who have serial seizures – that is, attacks which follow one after the other – or *status epilepticus,* or children with prolonged febrile convulsions, is in the form of diazepam suppositories (Stesolid). These are simple, effective and safe to give; they are placed in the rectum with an applicator. If someone in a family has frequent seizures their doctor may give them a supply of these suppositories so that they are on hand for emergency use.

A recent court case in Australia shows what a useful treatment this is felt to be. Stesolids are not licensed in Australia, although they are available. A physician who was treating patients in the outback was held to be at fault for not prescribing Stesolids for their emergency treatment, even though the drug was not licensed.

CLONAZEPAM (RIVOTRIL)

Clonazepam is also one of the benzodiazepine group of drugs, which are often used as tranquilizers. Its main value is its ability to control myoclonic seizures. It is also sometimes used as an alternative to Valium to control *status epilepticus*. It is usually given once daily (at night) although it is sometimes given twice a day, and its main drawback is that it has a strong sedative effect and causes drowsiness. Clonazepam will not be prescribed if your work requires you to be vigilant and alert. It may also cause personality changes, and these can, in my experience, be quite severe. One patient of mine changed from being a normal, affectionate teenager to an aggressive, rebellious tearaway; another attempted suicide soon after starting taking the drug. It is worth bearing this in mind if you notice that someone in your family who is taking the drug seems to be showing some personality change. See your doctor immediately because they will probably want to withdraw the drug straight away.

Another disadvantage of clonazepam, and of clobazam (a similar drug, see below) is that in some people tolerance develops fairly quickly, usually after three to six months. The drug then no longer has as great an effect. When tolerance has developed you will have to stop taking the drug for a while. However, even after a 'drug holiday' you may never regain the same response to the drug. With both clonazepam and clobazam you may get withdrawal effects when you stop taking it. These are the opposite of the tranquilizing effects; you may feel on edge all the time, anxious and 'twitchy', your skin my feel super-sensitive and you will be more sensitive to noise. These effects may last for one to three weeks.

When to avoid
Clonazepam should not be taken with alcohol, during pregnancy or if you are breast-feeding. If you are taking this drug and thinking of becoming pregnant you should talk to your doctor, because there is now evidence that clonazepam may lead to an unusually high percentage of fetal abnormalities. If you find that you are pregnant while taking clonazepam it is important to see your doctor immediately and discuss the implications with them. You will need to decide whether or not you wish to continue with the pregnancy (see pp.193–8).

CLOBAZAM (FRISIUM)

Clobazam, like clonazepam, is a benzodiazepine, but it seldom causes personality change and has a less marked sedative action than clonazepam. It is used to control both partial and generalized seizures, and is sometimes given as a supplementary drug to women who have catamenial epilepsy (see p.189). Its main success is in the reduction of partial complex seizures, and it has become very popular for treating these. Clobazam must be taken three times a day, and its main side-effect (seen mainly in large doses) is tiredness. Tolerance to the drug may also develop, with withdrawal effects when it is then stopped (see *Clonazepam*, above).

When to avoid
Clobazam should not be taken during pregnancy or if you are breast-feeding, and it should not be taken with alcohol.

ACETAZOLAMINE (DIAMOX)

Acetazolamine is sometimes given as a supplementary drug to women who have catamenial epilepsy (see p.189). It is also used as a 'Third Line' drug, to be given to people who have clusters of seizures at the time of each cluster. Tolerance to the drug develops after some time. Acetazolamine is a diuretic (causes increased excretion of water) and so anyone who takes it for any length of time needs to have regular blood tests to make sure that their body chemistry is not being thrown out of balance by this loss of water. Acetazolamine is thought to work by making the cells more 'acid' but this has not yet been convincingly proved.

PHENOBARBITONE (LUMINAL)

Phenobarbitone is one of the oldest, really effective anticonvulsant drugs, and in many parts of the world is still the most widely-used treatment for epilepsy. It has several advantages: it is safe, for example, is as good as carbamazepine, phenytoin or valproate in controlling generalized tonic clonic seizures and partial seizures, and is the cheapest of all the anticonvulsants. Because it has a long half-life it also need only be given once a day. However, although it rarely produces serious side-effects, it is a strong sedative and can have a marked effect on mental processes. Some people are particularly sensitive to phenobarbitone and become mentally dull, drowsy and lethargic. If it is given to young children it can have the opposite effect, making them overactive and badly behaved. These effects mean that phenobarbitone is now rarely used if other drugs are available.

PRIMIDONE (MYSOLINE)

Primidone is an interesting drug. It is a weak anticonvulsant in its own right, and its major anticonvulsant action comes from the metabolism of primidone into phenobarbitone. It thus suffers from all the advantages and disadvantages of phenobarbitone. Because primidone has this dual anticonvulsant effect it is now generally agreed that there is little point in giving phenobarbitone, when by giving primidone you are giving two anticonvulsants instead of one. Thus, if cost is not an important issue, primidone (which is slightly more expensive) is probably the drug of choice where phenobarbitone would have been used. A few people, however, are sensitive to primidone but not to phenobarbitone.

State-of-the-art drugs

Two new drugs are now on the market which have been developed specifically to affect the amount of 'GABA' (a substance which decreases the excitability of the brain by inhibiting the transmission of electrical impulses within it). These are gabapentin and vigabatrin. Drugs which decrease brain excitability by other means are also in the pipeline and will be available within the next few years.

GABAPENTIN (NEURONTIN)

Gabapentin acts by dampening down the excitatory system of the brain, and its main use is to control partial complex seizures, though it can also be useful as an anticonvulsant for generalized seizures. Gabapentin is a good anticonvulsant, but its other big advantage is that it is very safe. It is probably impossible to overdose on gabapentin, because however much of the drug is in the stomach, only a limited amount is absorbed into the bloodstream. And unlike many other anticonvulsants, gabapentin does not interfere with any other drugs you may be taking. This is because it is not metabolized in the liver; whatever is absorbed is excreted unchanged by the kidneys.

Possible side-effects
- Tiredness and muscle fatigue
- Rash
- Poor balance

When to avoid
Gabapentin is still a new drug and we are still in the process of learning more about it. Until it has been around longer, and people have had more experience of it, gabapentin should not be taken during pregnancy.

VIGABATRIN (SABRIL)

Vigabatrin is another new drug, specially developed as an anticonvulsant, which makes the brain less excitable by boosting its inhibitory ('damping down') system. It does this by preventing the breakdown of the inhibitory neurotransmitter, GABA. It is a very good anticonvulsant for partial complex seizures.

Its main side-effects are rashes, drowsiness, and not feeling well. More seriously, there have been reports that some people become depressed either when taking vigabatrin or when the drug is withdrawn, and that a few develop more serious psychiatric symptoms. However, this association with psychiatric symptoms is still very much an open question; some studies of the drug have shown good effects, some bad. Most doctors value vigabatrin as a useful addition to the drug armoury.

TOPIRAMATE (TOPRAMAX)

Topiramate is a new drug just recently licensed for use in partial complex seizures. In clinical trials it was very successful, decreasing the number of seizures by half in 50 per cent of the patients. Its mode of action is not yet known completely, but it seems to affect both the excitatory and inhibitory systems of the brain and thus have a wider action than some other drugs. Although it is still early days, so far it does not seem to have many undesirable side-effects.

'WONDER DRUGS'

Every now and then new 'wonder drugs' come onto the market in a blaze of publicity, guaranteed to provide the maximum of seizure control with the minimum of side-effects. These drugs are promoted enthusiastically by their manufacturers, but greeted by doctors who treat epilepsy with a mixture of hope and caution. One or two almost live up to their initial heady promise; most are eventually recognized as the usual combination of good news and bad news and take their place alongside all the other drugs in the epilepsy armoury. A few are hurriedly withdrawn as some unforeseen or unpredicted side-effect makes it apparent that they carry a risk which outweighs their benefits. Occasionally, too, there are drug-scare stories in the media leading to a condemnation of one particular drug.

Whatever the hype, your doctor will be influenced largely by how the drug *you* are taking affects *you*. If you have achieved good seizure control and have no serious side-effects your doctor probably will not suggest changing your medication.

FOLIC ACID

Some anticonvulsants reduce the level of folic acid in the blood. Folic acid deficiency can have serious consequences: anaemia, changes in the nervous system and, in a pregnant woman, spina bifida in the developing child. If you are taking phenobarbitone, phenytoin or primidone your doctor will therefore suggest that you take folic acid supplements by mouth. Unfortunately folic acid is also known to increase the brain's excitability and so tends to cause seizures, so it is possible that these supplements may give you a mild increase in seizure frequency. This is one of those 'swings and roundabouts' situations people with epilepsy so often have to face, but in this case the consequences of folic acid deficiency are serious enough to make it worth while putting up with a few more seizures.

You and your doctor

Epilepsy is a long-term condition, and epilepsy does not stand still. The character of your seizures may change and your drugs may need to be altered. You will be seeing your doctor regularly over the coming months and maybe even years, so it is important that you have a good relationship with them: one in which you can ask questions, ask for reassurance and get practical advice.

Once you've been diagnosed as having epilepsy, your follow-up may be in the hands of your GP or of a hospital consultant. If you are lucky you may be referred to a specialized epilepsy clinic, run by a neurologist or neuropsychiatrist with a special interest in epilepsy (see Appendix). The advantage of an epilepsy clinic is that it has a multidisciplinary team and can offer help not only with the medical aspects of epilepsy but with the social and psychological problems which people with epilepsy sometimes have to deal with too. They provide very good care, but unfortunately there are far too few of them around.

WHAT TO EXPECT FROM YOUR DOCTOR

- That they see you frequently and give you blood tests whenever you are started on a new drug.
- That he or she listens to what you have to say.
- That you are given regular check-ups, at least two every year, and ideally about once every three months.
- That you are given regular serum checks to check the level of drug in your blood and make sure your drug dosage is correct.

If your doctor fails to do these checks at least once a year (ideally more often), change to a doctor who does. *Do not* just carry on getting repeat prescriptions.

WHAT YOUR DOCTOR CAN EXPECT FROM YOU

- Keep on taking the tablets. It really is important that you take your medication regularly, just as it is prescribed. Failure to do this may mean that you will get withdrawal seizures. It may be safer not to take medication at all than to take it irregularly. Stick to your proper drug regime.
- Keep your appointments with the clinic or your doctor, and if you can't keep an appointment, *let them know.*

Becoming fit free

Anticonvulsant drugs work very well. They may have worked so well for you that you have not had a single seizure for two years or more. In that case you no longer have epilepsy, because epilepsy is defined as the occurrence of two or more seizures within a period of two years. So can you at last give up taking anticonvulsant drugs?

For someone who has had to take anticonvulsant medication every day of their life, maybe for years on end, coming off their drugs can seem like coming out of prison. It is the ultimate goal of treatment. And yet for adults, this is not an easy decision to make. There is always a small risk that when anticonvulsant drugs are stopped, seizures *may* recur, and if they do, control will be harder to re-establish. Secondly, there is a risk that withdrawal of the drug may itself cause a seizure, and if this happens you will be unable to drive for one year, even if you have no other seizure during this time (see *Epilepsy and driving*, pp.136–8).

If you have had no fits for two to three years, discuss the risks and benefits of giving up drugs with your doctor. What they advise will depend partly on how easily your seizures came under control in the first place. If, when your seizures first began, you immediately became seizure-free when you were put on drugs, there is a very good chance that your fits will not recur once your medication is stopped. Then it makes good sense to gradually reduce your drugs after two or three years, and perhaps eventually tail them off completely. However, if your seizures proved more difficult to control in the first place, then you are running more of a risk if you stop taking anticonvulsant medication. The seizures may start again, and if they do, there is no guarantee that they will be brought under control so successfully again. You will have to decide whether the benefits of giving up your drugs make this a risk you are prepared to run.

For children, the risk of seizures starting again after anticonvulsants have been withdrawn is rather less. In most children who have taken anticonvulsants for two years or more and been seizure-free, drugs can be withdrawn without the risk of seizures recurring. Two years after stopping treatment, three-quarters of children will still be seizure-free.

Outlook

Approximately one-third of all those people who develop epilepsy will eventually grow out of the condition and become fit-free. A further third will find that their seizures become less frequent and less severe with treatment, and the final third will remain unchanged. But remember that these are overall figures: the outlook in any particular case depends on the cause of the epilepsy, the age of onset, and whether or not there is a family history of the disease. Temporal lobe epilepsy, for example, is one of the most difficult types to treat successfully. So too is epilepsy which is the result of severe brain damage or of some degenerative brain disease. But for those people who have straightforward epilepsy, uncomplicated by brain damage, the outlook is good. For example, 80 per cent of people whose fits start after the age of 25 can be successfully controlled by drugs.

If you develop epilepsy during childhood and have a strong family history of the disease, there is an excellent chance that your epilepsy will improve after adolescence, or even that you will outgrow it altogether. This is because you have probably inherited the genes that increase the brain's excitability, and the effect of these genes decreases with age. Most children who have absences, for example, grow out of them by the age of 16.

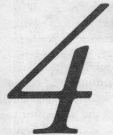

Chapter Four

Surgery for Epilepsy

*G*illian had had partial complex seizures since she started primary school. Now she was 16 and about to have temporal lobe surgery. Even as a child she had felt her epilepsy was a barrier between her and other people, making it hard for her to make friends. Now, at 16, she spent all her time at home and never went out. Although she didn't seem to mind this, her parents minded for her, especially her mother. "You'll see, everything will be different after your operation," her mother used to say. "You'll be able to go out, have boyfriends, be just like other girls."

The operation was a huge success. Gillian's parents were delighted (as well they might be – they had cashed in an insurance policy and had it done privately so that Gillian wouldn't have to wait) and so was her doctor. "We'll need to tail your drugs off gradually for a few months," he told her, "but then I don't see why you shouldn't stop altogether. Fingers crossed of course, but I think we can hope for a 100 per cent cure."

Two months later Gillian had had no seizures. But she had no social life either. She showed no signs of wanting to leave home or lead an independent life. "You can't just keep on sitting at home now," said her mother. "Come on, we've paid all that money for your operation so you could start leading a proper life of your own. You should start going out, meeting people, making friends . . ."

But Gillian had never learnt how to make friends. With people of her own age she felt out of her depth. She didn't know how to talk to them, she didn't share their interests. In her heart of hearts she knew she didn't really want to get to know them – she was scared. Her epilepsy didn't seem like a barrier any more, more like a protective wall around her which had been suddenly demolished.

The next day Gillian didn't take her anticonvulsants. She didn't take them next day, or the day after that. A few days later she had a seizure. Her parents of course were bitterly disappointed. So was Gillian, in a way . . . but there was a part of her, quite a large part in fact, which felt as though she was welcoming back an old friend.

It is only within the last few years that surgery has been a serious option for someone with epilepsy. The first brain operations tended to be rather hit-or-miss affairs. But modern methods of brain imaging mean that the surgeon can pinpoint the area of the brain which is giving rise to seizures much more accurately and brain surgery is much safer and more successful (and therefore more popular and widely used) than it used to be. The surgeon now knows exactly which part of the brain has to be removed, and can predict much more easily which people will benefit from surgery and what the effects of surgery are likely to be.

Even so, epilepsy surgery is not something to be gone into lightly. It will only be considered if drug treatment has failed. Not every patient will benefit from surgery, not every type of seizure will be improved. You will have to be prepared for months of tests – and you also have to be prepared for disappointment. Each further test is a hurdle at which you may fall.

If epilepsy surgery is being offered to children, it is important for the whole family to be assessed and to know what is involved. Parents who are desperate for a cure for their child may put undue pressure on them to have surgery. And they may also have unrealistic expectations about what surgery can achieve. There can be problems if parents (like Gillian's parents) expect that the operation will change their child overnight. It will not suddenly give him or her the social skills they need to make friends, for example.

Even the loss of seizures can be a mixed blessing. For a few people their seizures are very much a part of their identity. They may find it hard to come to terms with their loss; in fact, losing their seizures may actually be more traumatic for them at the time than the continuation of their epilepsy. Although children will have experienced the down side of having epilepsy, they may also have grown used to being dependent or to having attention lavished upon them. A new, seizure-free life style may not be entirely welcome if it means they are expected to become independent and allowances are no longer made for them.

There is one question which often worries people who are thinking about epilepsy surgery. One might expect the operation itself to damage the brain and give rise to even more seizures, and yet this does not happen. The reason is that although the clean cut of the surgeon's knife (provided it is skillfully wielded) obviously damages some cells, the damage is limited and local and usually not sufficient for seizures to arise.

WHO BENEFITS?

Before anyone considers you as a candidate for surgery, you will be put through a whole battery of tests to see if surgery would be likely to abolish or at least reduce the frequency of your seizures. The surgeon also needs to make sure that the surgery itself would not be likely to cause any further damage. You are most likely to benefit from epilepsy surgery:

- If you have partial complex seizures due to temporal lobe epilepsy;
- If it is quite clear which side of the brain the seizures are coming from;
- If you do not have a 'mix' of seizures (i.e., all your seizures are of one type);

- If your seizures arise from a single, localized focus;
- If this focus is in a part of the brain which can be easily removed without causing significant impairment of brain function, or damage to other structures;

Assessment tests

You will have to undergo at least some of the following ranges of tests to check whether you are a good candidate for surgery.

- A detailed clinical history is the first and most important check. From it your doctor can usually ensure that you only have one seizure type, and deduce the likely area of the brain from which your seizures are arising.
- Routine and sleep EEGs will indicate whether your seizures appear to arise from a localized focus (see p.31).
- Sphenoidal EEG recording, foramen ovale recording or videotelemetry (pp.32–3), to check which side and which part of the temporal lobe seizures are coming from.
- MRI scan (pp.33–6). This gives more accurate information about the origin of your seizures and whether the damage is confined to one side of the brain.
- PET scan and SPET (p.38). These give a picture of the brain at work, and are used to confirm that the lesion is on a particular side. If there is a lesion it will show up on the scan as a zone of low metabolism (i.e., low brain activity).
- Psychometric tests (pp.36–8). These will give additional evidence about the focus of the seizures, and also indicate whether your memory or other mental processes would be likely to suffer as a result of an operation.

Temporal lobe surgery

The people most likely to benefit from epilepsy surgery are those who have seizures which arise in the temporal lobe. The operation usually involves removal of the front 3–6 cm of the lobe. However, if your seizures arise from a tumour or from one specific area of damage tissue, the surgeon will perform a 'lumpectomy' or a 'lesionectomy', removing only this particular tissue.

Success of temporal lobe surgery

Temporal lobe surgery almost always reduces the frequency and severity of seizures. About 80 per cent of people who have the operation are much improved and about 50 per cent lose their seizures altogether. The people who do best are those who had febrile convulsions as children and now have damage to a small area, the hippocampus, deep inside the temporal lobe. Where there is damage to the outside of the temporal lobe following an infection such as meningitis or a head injury, surgery is usually less successful.

A decrease in seizure frequency is not the only benefit of surgery. Many people find that the operation often improves their quality of life in other ways; some are able to return to work, some report that the quality of their sex lives has improved. Parents whose children have had the operation often say that it has made them less difficult – their behaviour is better and they are less aggressive. Children will often start to do better at school and the loss of their seizures may increase their confidence and social ability.

Those are the benefits. What about the risks? Anyone who is thinking about epilepsy surgery has to take into account the fact that *any* brain surgery involves risks and epilepsy surgery is no different. About one in a hundred people who have epilepsy surgery will suffer some serious damage: paralysis of an arm or leg, or some loss of speech if the operation is on the side of the brain where speech occurs. Yet there is no way of predicting whether this damage will happen in any individual case.

Although doctors can predict quite accurately which patients are likely to lose their seizures after surgery, it is not nearly so easy to predict how it will affect their behaviour and personality. Any major surgery is a major life-event, and so it is not too surprising that a few people suffer a depressive illness after surgery. A few people (about 0.4 per cent) develop a more serious, schizophrenia-like illness after temporal lobe surgery. But there is no real evidence that this is linked specifically to the operation; it is more likely that these are people who might have developed the illness anyway. There is some evidence that this illness happens more often when the operation is on the right side. Memory is also often affected by temporal lobe surgery, and is likely to be more severely affected when the operation is on the left side.

SPHENOIDAL RECORDING

For a successful operation, there must be as accurate a 'fix' as possible on the damaged area. A normal EEG, in which the electrodes are simply attached to the scalp, can usually record abnormal activity going on deep in the brain, but it will not give a very clear indication of the exact area the activity is coming from. So before you have temporal lobe surgery, you may be given a special kind of EEG, called a sphenoidal recording, to pinpoint the area of the temporal lobe which is giving rise to seizures.

A sphenoidal EEG recording is usually carried out in an operating theatre. The electrodes are inserted just above the angle of the jaws, so that they lie just outside the skull on each side but as close as possible to the deeper part of the temporal lobes. An injection of a general anaesthetic is then given, in an attempt to induce abnormal EEG activity. If epileptic spikes are seen, it is possible to tell which side of the brain they are arising from, and whether they are coming from the deeper part of the temporal lobe or from the surface. Often one anaesthetic agent may not be enough to induce abnormal EEG activity, so two or three injections may be given with different anaesthetics before the patient is allowed to recover fully.

If you have to have this procedure, be prepared for the insertion of the wires to be slightly painful. In children the anaesthetic is given first, before the wires are inserted. This is not ideal because if possible the EEG should be measured immediately the anaesthetic is given, before the brain has had time to become accustomed to it. Adults are therefore expected to put up with the discomfort during insertion.

In some units the sphenoidal wires are kept in place for several days. During this time patients return to the ward and are monitored continuously (see *Telemetry* pp.32–3). To begin with, the wires may make chewing slightly painful, but this soon settles down and after a day or so you do not know that they are in.

FORAMEN OVALE ELECTRODES

In some units a different kind of recording is carried out to discover exactly where in the temporal lobe the seizures are coming from. In this procedure electrodes are inserted actually inside the skull so that they lie outside the brain but right alongside its surface. However, now that other modern imaging techniques are available, foramen ovale electrodes are used much less often than they were.

The patient is given a general anaesthetic and under X-ray control an electrode is pushed into each cheek and then angled upwards so that they pass through a small oval hole (called the foramen ovale) on each side in the base of the skull. The electrodes come to lie along the medial surface of the temporal lobe, close to the hippocampus.

The electrodes are left in place until you have a seizure, on average for about five days. If after two days you have had no seizures, your drugs will be reduced to encourage seizures to occur.

For the first two days after the electrodes have been inserted, the cheeks are sore and swollen and you feel rather like a hamster. You may also notice changes in sensation in the face, because the nerve which supplies sensation to the face also passes through the foramen ovale. But this soon settles down and most people say the procedure is not *too* unpleasant. The electrodes are removed while you are awake, but this is not usually painful.

DEPTH ELECTRODES

Sometimes even with detailed neuroimaging or foramen ovale telemetry it is still not possible to be certain which temporal lobe is giving rise to seizures. In this case it may be necessary to put electrodes right inside the brain to record seizure activity.

These intracranial electrodes are either special EEG electrodes which can be placed on the brain's surface or thin electrode wires which can be inserted through the substance of the brain so that they lie close to the areas from which seizures are thought to be arising.

Insertion of these 'depth electrodes' is a complicated procedure and can only be done in units which have special facilities. The patient is given a general anaesthetic, and holes are drilled in their skull through which both brain surface electrodes and indwelling brain electrodes are inserted. This is all done using special equipment so the surgeon knows exactly where the electrodes are being inserted.

The patient then returns to the ward and is monitored (see telemetry pp.32–3) for one to two weeks until a number of seizures have been recorded and their point of onset has been determined. For the first few days after the electrode insertion some patients are confused and disorientated and so they are nursed in a neurosurgical ward.

BRAIN STIMULATION

It is not only the seizure area that has to be mapped out before epilepsy surgery. There is always a small risk that adjacent areas might be damaged and so it is important to know if this adjacent damage might lead to any serious loss of brain function. In the case of temporal lobe surgery the most vulnerable area is usually the speech area – the so-called 'eloquent' cortex. In the frontal lobe it is the area which controls movement – the 'motor cortex'.

Depth electrodes are one way of finding out exactly where this vulnerable area is. Once the indwelling or surface electrodes are in place and the patient has recovered from the anaesthetic, each electrode can be stimulated in turn with a very small current. Those electrodes whose stimulation interferes with speech (or any other function) will be noted. This allows the surgeon to map the vulnerable area very precisely and avoid it at operation.

Weighing up the risks

There is always some risk in opening the skull and putting wires into or onto the surface of the brain. No surgeon will suggest such invasive procedures unless it is thought the benefits will outweigh the potential risks. So the use of depth electrodes will only be considered if your epilepsy is so severe that you cannot live a reasonable life, and other brain imaging methods have failed to locate the source of your seizures. Sometimes it is a risk worth taking, but you should always discuss it with your doctor.

Frontal lobe surgery

Frontal lobe seizures are very resistant to drug treatment and so people with this type of epilepsy are often considered for surgery. But just as with temporal lobe surgery, they will have to be carefully assessed first of all to make sure they are suitable candidates for surgery.

If the seizures are all arising from the frontal lobe and the MRI scan shows that there is a lesion, then two operations can be done. The first is to remove only the lesion in the hope that this will stop the seizures. The second option is to remove a large chunk of the frontal lobe (frontal lobectomy). This is the operation that is usually done if the lesion is large.

If no lesion is found on the MRI scan, the next step will be to insert depth electrodes (see p.69) while the patient is under a general anaesthetic. Leashes of thin electrode wires are inserted into the frontal lobe through a burr hole in the skull. These are kept in place for one to two weeks, and the EEG activity from them is measured continuously, until enough seizures have been captured to make it clear where they are arising. If they are arising from a single epileptic focus, even though its exact size is uncertain this focus may be removed by taking away a large area of frontal lobe surrounding the focus.

Success of frontal lobe surgery

Frontal lobe surgery is not usually as successful as temporal lobe surgery. If an actual lesion is found by MRI scanning and removed, about 40 per cent of people who have the operation will lose their seizures. If, on the other hand, the MRI shows no clear structural lesion although the EEG shows that there is a focus from which seizures are arising, only between 20 and 30 per cent of patients having the operation will lose their seizures. Unfortunately removal of a frontal lobe often causes personality changes, and this is something that anyone who is considering the operation should discuss in detail with their doctor before making a final decision to go ahead.

Hemispherectomy

Hemispherectomy is an operation to remove one half (or hemisphere) of the brain, either partly or completely. Clearly, this is heroic surgery, and it will only be carried out if the hemisphere is already so badly damaged that the person is intensely disabled by it.

71

Sometimes this kind of extensive damage is caused by an infection such as encephalitis. Often the damage occurs either during development in the womb or around the time of birth. The baby is born with one half of his or her brain so badly damaged that seizures arise in it continually. These continual seizures are not only very disabling in themselves, but they may prevent the other half of the brain developing normally. The child may be weak or paralysed on one side of their body (hemiplegic) and have a loss of one half of the field of vision in each eye. Often the child is very difficult and aggressive and has other severe behaviour problems too.

Sometimes the only way to help these children is to remove the damaged half of the brain altogether. However, this is an operation that will only be considered if the child already has severe brain damage, and the brain damage is confined to one side of the brain.

One way of performing this operation is to remove the damaged hemisphere altogether, leaving the tough outer covering of the brain (the dura) and attaching this to the midline to fill in the gap left after removing the brain tissue. Another (called the Montreal technique, because the method was developed there) is to leave the hemisphere in place, but to cut all the nerve connections from it. The blood supply is left intact, so that what is left is essentially a live, but totally inactive, hemisphere.

Success of hemispherectomy
All young children who are given this operation already have severe learning difficulties, with some degree of hemiplegia (paralysis of one half of the body) and are very dependent. The operation will not alter these disabilities. But many do have a much better quality of life after the operation. Parents often notice that their child's behaviour improves and that they become less aggressive. Because they have fewer or even no seizures the child's medication can usually be reduced, and this in itself will make them brighter and more responsive.

Callosotomy

Another type of operation is sometimes considered for someone who has very severe epilepsy in which the seizures arise all over the brain and cause 'drop attacks' (see p.10) during which they may be badly hurt. This is callosotomy, an operation to cut, either partially or completely, the nerve tracts (corpus callosum) that connect the two halves of the brain. Occasionally the operation is also offered to people with severe partial complex seizures.

Usually about a third of the corpus callosum is cut to begin with. If this does not prove successful, another third of the fibres will be cut, and finally a total split may be made.

Success of callosotomy

Callosotomy will not end the seizures, but it will change their nature. The operation will stop the seizures spreading from one side of the brain to the other, which in turn will help prevent the drop attacks. Between 65 and 100 per cent of patients have at least a 50 per cent reduction in drop attacks, rising to nearer 100 per cent some time after the operation.

Some patients are mute for a few days after the operation, but, perhaps surprisingly, it has been found that full callosotomy proves to be no more of a disadvantage to the patient than partial callosotomy. There may be some unwanted effects, for example a lack of co-ordination between the two hands.

The right age to operate

The age at which you have epilepsy surgery usually depends on the type of lesion you have. Obviously, if seizures are caused by a malignant tumour this will be removed, if possible, as soon as it is discovered. But if the surgery is only for epilepsy, there is no urgency; it can be done whenever it is convenient for you.

Most surgery involves lesions in the temporal lobe, and here the age at operation does seem to make a difference to its success. It used to be thought that there was no advantage in carrying out surgery early, and that it was better for the patient to wait until he or she was adult. But now it is believed that on the whole, the earlier temporal lobe surgery is carried out, the better. People who have the operation before puberty are more likely to be able to give up their drugs completely after it, and less likely to suffer any subsequent deterioration, so that they will have a more normal personality and be more independent. It is not yet known whether early operation is an advantage for people who have frontal lobe seizures but it is likely that it may be.

However, age is no barrier to operation, and here again, thinking has changed. Neurosurgeons used to believe that it was not advisable to perform temporal lobe surgery on anyone over 40. The view now taken is that one can operate up to almost any age, though the older the patient the more hazardous the operation becomes.

5

Alternative Approaches to Seizure Control

D rugs are the most widely used and, for most people, the most effective way of controlling seizures. But they are not the only way, and they do not help everybody. If no conventional drug treatment seems to have much effect on the frequency or severity of your seizures, it is worth trying a more unorthodox approach as well. However, this should not be your *only* form of treatment if you have frequent seizures. Even if anticonvulsant drugs work well for you, you may be able to improve your seizure control still more by using one of these complementary methods.

Anything that affects your own attitude of mind or makes you feel better or happier is likely to improve your seizure control. And so, although there is no real scientific evidence that, say, faith healing or acupuncture or hypnosis can influence seizures, if you feel you would like to try them they may very well work for *you*. Certainly they will have no harmful effects.

It is worth considering an alternative approach to seizure control if:

- You have no warning (aura) that a seizure is starting and so cannot use many of the self-help measures discussed on pp.93–110;

75

- Your seizures are poorly controlled by drugs alone.

If you are interested in trying any of the alternative approaches to seizure control discussed below, get in touch with the British Epilepsy Association (see Appendix) who will help you contact the appropriate centre.

Biofeedback

In 1964 Barry Sterman, a research worker in California, was working on a NASA contract looking at the toxic effects of the rocket fuel hydrazine. He had been asked by NASA to feed this fuel to cats and see whether or not it affected the cats' nervous systems.

Hydrazine is known to be a convulsant (i.e., to cause seizures), and so Sterman was not surprised to discover that, when he fed this fuel to cats, some had seizures. What was much more surprising was that one group of cats did *not* have seizures. For some reason they seemed remarkably resistant to the convulsant effects of the fuel.

What was so special about these particular cats? In an effort to find out, Sterman decided to look more closely at their previous history. He discovered that they had all taken part in another experiment that he was conducting in his laboratory. The cats had had EEG electrodes fixed to their heads so that their brain activity could be measured. They had then been 'conditioned' to see whether they were able to modify their own brain activity.

Barry Sterman was particularly interested in a brain rhythm which was generated over the sensorimotor cortex, that area of the brain which deals with the control of movement, and so the cats had been conditioned to increase sensorimotor activity.

Whenever they did so (purely by chance at first) they were rewarded by being given a saucer of milk. Gradually they learned that a particular behaviour invariably led to the reward of milk. What the cats learned to do was simply to remain absolutely still. It was this immobility that led to an increase in the brain rhythm. And Sterman believed that somehow this increase in the sensorimotor rhythm was protecting the cats from the convulsant effects of the hydrazine rocket fuel.

If cats could learn to modify their brain rhythms, Sterman argued, then why should humans not learn to do it too? If an increase in the sensorimotor rhythm did indeed act as an anticonvulsant, then people who had epilepsy might also be taught to increase this particular brain rhythm, and so possibly reduce their seizure frequency.

Seeing the brain's activity

Sterman then tried the experiment on people with epilepsy. EEG electrodes were attached to the subject's head to record the brain's electrical waves, or rhythms. These rhythms were first amplified in the EEG machine, and then filtered to select the particular rhythms the subject was trying to modify. Next, these electrical waves were fed into a computer which drove a light display, designed so that if there was any increase in the selected rhythm, the lights moved across the screen. The person could actually see the activity of their brain in visual form, as the light moved across the display. This is called biofeedback (literally, to be made aware of some aspect of body function of which one is normally not conscious).

The subjects were then 'trained' by being told to try to make the lights move across the board. They had to find their own method of doing this, by searching for some 'mind activity' or act of will which would move the lights in the right direction.

Sterman found that some patients could indeed modify their brain rhythms and that the exercise did help them to control their seizures. In his first trial a number of patients were able to decrease the frequency of their seizures by well over half. Some found that, like the cats, they could do so by sitting still. Others discovered different strategies, and some were highly successful but could not say just how they managed to do it. Like the cats, the patients were rewarded, though not with milk. They were given tokens which could be exchanged for sweets or money every time their brain activity was increased (i.e., the lights moved) beyond a certain point.

Once Sterman had shown that people could learn to reduce their seizure frequency by modifying brain activity, other laboratories were inspired to try similar experiments to see whether there were other anticonvulsant brain rhythms. Many people have fewer seizures when they are alert, and so one of the obvious targets for biofeedback training was to teach people to increase the brain rhythms which occur when you are alert. This was found to be equally successful. People with epilepsy usually have an increase of slow rhythms in their brains, and so people were taught to use biofeedback to reduce this slow activity. It was found that this exercise too helped to reduce seizures.

OTHER BIOFEEDBACK METHODS

Other biofeedback methods make use of a slightly different principle. One of the first investigators was Schwab in the 1950s who argued that if people could be stimulated at the onset of a seizure, then the seizure could be avoided. He put EEG electrodes on people who had absence seizures. When they had an absence seizure, the EEG recorded spike waves and, as it did so, a light bulb would flash. The flash alerted the person and this shortened the attacks. Eventually the person learned to alert themselves at the beginning of a seizure, without the stimulus of the flashing light. It was hoped that this method would stop the attacks altogether, but this result has never been achieved.

Other workers have shown that biofeedback can be used to teach patients to detect the abnormal electrical discharges – the spikes of epilepsy – which occur between seizures, and to reduce them. Reducing the spikes should also lead to a reduction in seizure frequency. This method too has been quite successful and helped a number of people to achieve a reduction in their seizure frequency.

We tried this method of seizure control at the Maudsley Hospital, and found that we could indeed teach people to reduce their spikes. It then occurred to us that if people could learn to decrease their spikes, maybe they could also learn to increase their spikes. In fact, perhaps the number of spikes that they have was to some extent under their control. We found that this was indeed the case. People were able to increase the number of spikes in their EEG in the same way as they can be taught to decrease them.

This result was interesting in itself, but something even more interesting emerged from the study. We found that many people, once they recognized that their spike numbers were increasing, refused to continue with the experiment. The reason they gave was that they recognized that they had to stop putting a 'mental brake' on their seizures. In other words, they acknowledged that they already had special mental 'tricks' for keeping their seizures under control, and to stop these tricks would allow their seizures to increase. This was a startling finding, as it suggested that, to some extent, people can modify their own seizures, and can do so by modifying the way they think, and how they behave. These ideas now form the basis for yet another drug-free method of treating epilepsy – the behavioural treatment described in Chapter 6.

Recently, Professor Niels Birbaumer, from Tübingen in Germany, has used biofeedback in a rather different way. It has been known for some time that the cortex becomes more excitable when it is electrically negatively charged. It therefore seemed possible that if the cortex were made more positive and therefore *less* excitable, seizures would be less likely to occur. Birbaumer did this using biofeedback.

The experiment he devised was very similar to Barry Sterman's. Special electrodes were fixed to the scalp and connected to an EEG machine. The output of the EEG machine was interfaced with a computer, which could measure the amount of negativity or positivity. The display on the computer screen showed a space ship, which moved off its launch pad when the subject managed to make his cortex positive. The more positive the cortex, the further the space ship moved; the aim was to try and get it right off its launch pad and across to the other side of the computer screen.

After some training, most people were able to produce this positivity at will, and they were then instructed to practise at home without the help of the machine. Finally, once they had demonstrated that they knew how to achieve increased positivity and could do it easily, they were told to do it whenever they were in a situation in which they knew from experience that a seizure was likely to occur, or, if they had an aura, right at the beginning of a seizure. This kind of biofeedback training is still in its infancy, but certainly some of the people in research trials who have practised it say that it has greatly reduced their seizure frequency.

There is no doubt that biofeedback training in general can help to reduce seizure frequency, and that it might be especially valuable in people who have severe epilepsy which does not respond to medication. So why has this effective, drug-free method of treatment never really caught on? Unfortunately the reasons are very clear. Like so many things, it is a question of time and money. Biofeedback training is very time-consuming. It takes about 10 to 16 hour-long training sessions to learn the technique, as well as regular practice sessions at home. The patient must be highly motivated, and the training team very dedicated. And although the equipment itself is not very expensive, you do have to have a laboratory to put it in and a clinical psychologist to run the programme. Sadly, it seems that biofeedback requires a great deal more energy and commitment than most epilepsy services, or indeed most epilepsy sufferers, are able or willing to give. But if you are happy to work at it, it is a method worth considering.

Relaxation

If you are one of the many people who tend to get more seizures when they are under stress, learning to relax may prove to be a very effective way of reducing the frequency of your seizures. Almost any relaxation technique can be helpful. It is something you can teach yourself at home, using either a special relaxation tape, or following the instructions in the method given below. If you prefer, you may be able to join a relaxation class where you can learn in a group. Once you have learnt a relaxation technique, you can try using it whenever you feel that a seizure seems imminent, or you are in a seizure-prone situation.

Learning to relax
When you are learning physical relaxation, choose a time to practise when you are not feeling too tense; at first you will find it a difficult technique to master unless you are feeling fairly relaxed to start with. Find a quiet room where you will not be interrupted and are away from distractions.

You can either sit or lie down, whichever is the most comfortable for you. Make sure that your arms and legs are not crossed and that you are sitting or lying square. Close your eyes. It often helps to have some relaxing music on as a background.

I To begin with, just concentrate on your breathing. Breathe through your nose with a slow even rhythm for a few minutes. Try to breathe from your diaphragm, not from your chest. Now take a deep breath in and hold it for two seconds. As you breathe out, say 'Relax' out loud. Continue these slow deep breaths five or six times, each time saying the word 'Relax' as you breathe out.

In time you will be able to think the word 'Relax' in your mind. Now you are going to use this same rhythm of breathing as you learn to relax each of your body parts in turn.

2 First, clench both your fists tightly together for about ten seconds. As you do so breathe in, hold your breath and feel the tension in your fists and fingers. Then relax your fists and breathe out, thinking the word 'Relax'. Feel the difference between tension and relaxation. Do this twice.

3 Now bring your forearms towards your shoulders, tensing them up as you do so and breathing in. Hold the position for about ten seconds. Then breathe out, saying 'Relax' to yourself. Feel the difference between tension and relaxation. Repeat.

4 Now your shoulders. Shrug both your shoulders towards your ears. Breathe in and feel the tension as you do so. Hold the position for ten seconds. Breathe out, saying 'Relax' and feeling the difference between tension and relaxation. Repeat.

5 Bend your right ear down towards your shoulder, feeling the tension along the side of your neck. (Try not to lift your shoulder up towards your ear.) Again, breathe in as you do so, hold the position for ten seconds, then breathe out and think 'Relax', bringing your head back up. Repeat this exercise and then do the same thing twice with your left ear.

6 Now bring your chin down to your chest, feeling the tension at the back of your neck and breathing in as you do so. Hold it there for ten seconds, then breathe out saying 'Relax', and bring your head upright. Repeat.

7 Now try to tense and relax the muscles of your face. Screw up your eyes and purse your lips together. Again, breathe in as you do so, hold the position for ten seconds, then relax and breathe out. Feel the difference between tension and relaxation. Repeat.

At this point go over your body in your mind's eye and check that your arms and hands are relaxed, that your neck and shoulders are relaxed, and that your neck and face are relaxed. You may need to perform this check after each exercise, because tension creeps back in easily while you are concentrating on something else.

8 Relaxing your back muscles is the next step. Breathe in and as you do so hollow your back, pushing your spine forwards so that you can feel the tension along your back. Hold it for ten seconds, then breathe out and relax. Feel the difference between tension and relaxation. Repeat.

9 Next pull your stomach muscles in, breathing in as you do, so that there is tension all the way across your stomach like an elastic band tightening around your waist. Then breathe out and relax. Repeat.

10 Now tense your buttocks by clenching them together, breathing in as you do so. Keep them clenched for ten seconds. Now breathe out and relax, feeling the difference between tension and relaxation. Repeat.

11 To relax your feet, if you are sitting, raise your legs and point your toes. If you are lying down, just point your toes. Breathe in as you do so and feel the tension along the tops and backs of your shins and calves. Breathe out and relax. Repeat.

12 Finally, tense and relax your thighs and your calves. Push your legs down into the ground as hard as you can, feeling the tension all the way along your legs. Hold the position for ten seconds. Breathe out and relax, feeling the difference between tension and relaxation. Repeat.

13 You have now relaxed each of the major muscle groups in your body. For the final few minutes of the exercise, sit or lie and concentrate on the music, pushing any worrying thoughts to the back of your mind. Check your body again in your mind's eye to make sure there are no bits of tension remaining. Keep your breathing slow and regular.

When you start to do this exercise it will take a while to get your body fully relaxed, but the more you practise, the easier it becomes. The next stage is to build the habit of relaxation into your everyday life. Every now and then during the day, stop what you are doing and just relax for a minute or two. You can do this quite quickly and unobtrusively.

Consolidating physical relaxation techniques

Now that you know the difference between tension and relaxation, and can relax your muscles at will, it is a good idea to check each part of your body occasionally during the day to see whether your muscles are tensed or relaxed. If you find some areas of tension, take a few slow deep breaths, then breathe out, relaxing those muscles as you do so.

When you have become used to physical relaxation and find it easy, you can use it when you find you are in seizure-prone situations or at seizure onset.

To begin with, at the end of each relaxation session it may help to imagine how you would use these new skills in seizure-prone situations. When you are fully relaxed:

1 Imagine a situation in which you are likely to have a seizure. Try to visualize it as clearly as you can – what you might be doing, feeling and thinking.
2 Now say to yourself, 'Relax', and physically relax your body at the same time as imagining relaxing in the setting you have visualized.
3 Now imagine you can continue with whatever you were doing before you felt a seizure might occur. Feel pleased with yourself for having been able to avoid a seizure by relaxing.

When you are using this imagination technique, it is often easier to start by imagining a situation in which you know you can sometimes stop a seizure arising, and gradually work up to imagining situations in which you feel you would have least control over the onset of the seizure. Make a list of seizure-prone situations ranking them from 'least likely' to 'most likely' to provoke a seizure (your ABC charts – see p.97 – will be helpful when you are doing this).

Practise the imagination exercise with each item on your list, starting with the 'least likely'. When you are able to feel quite relaxed as you imagine it, move on to the next item on your list, gradually working your way up until you are able to relax even while you are imagining your most seizure-prone situation.

You are now ready to start using these skills in seizure-prone situations in your everyday life. Even when you feel you have mastered the relaxation technique, it is a good idea to keep in practice by giving yourself a full relaxation session every now and then.

Relaxing the mind
True relaxation should involve the mind as well as the body. Practising the exercises described above will eventually help you to relax at will. But you will find the benefits increase considerably if you can also learn to calm your mind at the same time. A simple meditation or yoga practice can help you to do this (see p.92).

Covert desensitization

Once you have learnt to relax whenever you feel that you are in a seizure-prone situation, you can try another technique which uses relaxation to 'desensitize' you – that is, make you less anxious about the idea of having a seizure. Many people find that as they gradually become less anxious about the fact that they might have a seizure in the future, they seem to have fewer seizures. You will need a co-therapist if you try this exercise – someone who can talk you through the programme when you are practising it.

The first stage is to identify all the aspects of having a seizure that make you feel anxious. List these in order from the ones that cause you most anxiety (say, having a seizure in a crowded public place) to those that make you least anxious (say, having a seizure when you are relaxing at home with your family).

DESENSITIZING EXERCISE

Once you have your hierarchy of anxiety-provoking situations you are ready to start this exercise.

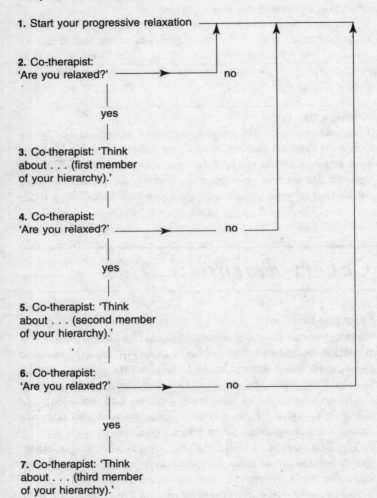

1. Start your progressive relaxation

2. Co-therapist:
'Are you relaxed?'   no

yes

3. Co-therapist: 'Think about . . . (first member of your hierarchy).'

4. Co-therapist:
'Are you relaxed?'   no

yes

5. Co-therapist: 'Think about . . . (second member of your hierarchy).'

6. Co-therapist:
'Are you relaxed?'   no

yes

7. Co-therapist: 'Think about . . . (third member of your hierarchy).'

At first, each time you practise you will probably find there is a sticking point at which you have to go back to the beginning and relax before starting again. But gradually, after a few sessions, you should find that you are able to think your way through the whole hierarchy without feeling tense.

Psychotherapy

Psychotherapy simply means talking to someone. Your doctor, if he is a good doctor, will give you psychotherapy every time you go and see him. But not every doctor has the time, and a few do not have the inclination or the skills to give patients who have epilepsy time to talk about the problems they have with their condition and the anxieties they feel. Individual psychotherapy on a one-to-one basis will give you the chance to have these discussions. Some GP practices have their own counsellor attached to the practice. If yours does not, ask your GP to refer you to a counselling service in your area.

Group support

Whether you have epilepsy yourself or are the parent of a child with epilepsy, it helps to have someone to talk to who understands your worries and concerns. Through your local branch of the British Epilepsy Association or your doctor, you may be able to join a group of other people who have epilepsy and their relatives. It can be very reassuring to be able to compare your experiences and talk about your anxieties to other people who know exactly what you mean, because they have probably gone through very similar experiences themselves.

Discussing problems you share can be helpful. You will find that other people have many of the same problems that you do, but they may have found ways of dealing with them that have not occurred to you. Knowing that other people have to deal with the same everyday problems or irritations of living with epilepsy can make you feel less isolated and bring your epilepsy more into perspective. This has a knock-on effect too; if you feel better adjusted and more relaxed about your epilepsy, the chances are that your seizures will start to occur less frequently.

Most of these groups meet regularly, sometimes socially, sometimes to hear a talk or have a discussion group. If there is no such group in your area, why not start one? Remember that one person in 200 has epilepsy. Wherever you are, there will be people who will want to join.

Videorecording

No one ever sees themselves during a seizure. Even if you have epilepsy yourself, you may never have seen anyone else have a seizure. Videorecording can be helpful if one of your main worries about having a seizure is what you look like, how you appear to onlookers and what they think of you. People who have been shown videotapes of their seizures during treatment sessions have found that they tend to have significantly fewer seizures afterwards. Imagination usually far outstrips reality, and what you see – the reality of what actually happens in a seizure – is probably much less disturbing than you had imagined it would be.

If you want to try this technique, you will again need a co-therapist with a video camera who spends enough time with you to make it likely that they will be around to capture a seizure on camera. Obviously it makes it much easier to arrange for them to be there at the right time if you know there are some situations in which you are especially likely to have a seizure.

Aromatherapy

Aromatherapy is a pioneering treatment for epilepsy. At present only one unit (The Seizure Clinic and Epilepsy Liaison Service at Birmingham University) offers it, but there is increasing interest in it and it may soon be more readily available in other epilepsy centres. At the very least it is a pleasant and totally safe treatment with no side-effects; at best there is a good chance that it may reduce your seizure frequency. A few people have even become seizure free using this method.

Aromatherapy may help you if you usually have a warning or aura before a seizure, and if you have kept a seizure diary so that you know the psychological state in which you are most likely to have a seizure – perhaps when you are very tense and anxious, for example.

You will be asked to choose an aromatherapy oil from a selection which are believed to have relaxing properties. You will then be taught how to relax, using a self-hypnosis technique, while at the same time sniffing the oil you have chosen. If you find it hard to relax, or are one of the many people who are in such a continual state of tension that you do not really recognize the difference between tension and relaxation, you will be given between three and six body massages with the oil. The smell of the oil will gradually become associated with the feeling of relaxation, and eventually the association becomes so strong that by simply sniffing the oil you will be able to make yourself relax.

Your seizure diary may show that you are one of the minority who actually have *more* seizures when they are relaxed. In this case you will be taught to develop a similar association between the smell of the oil and some technique for making yourself more alert and aroused.

Once you have learned the association, when you experience a warning aura, or know you are in a situation in which you are liable to have a seizure, sniffing your bottle of oil may be enough to abort it. A few people even develop a 'smell memory' for the oil so that they need only think about it to stop the seizure.

Do not try do-it-yourself aromatherapy, but find a properly trained aromatherapist. Pure aromatherapy oils must be used (some commercially-available ones, such as those from the Body Shop, will not do) and it is important to use the same brand all the time so that the smell is absolutely consistent. The choice of oil is important too; it has been suggested, though as yet the evidence is not conclusive, that some oils have anticonvulsant properties and may inhibit seizures. But there are others which can occasionally cause fits, so always consult an expert.

Acupuncture

Acupuncture is a branch of Chinese medicine, based on the belief that the life force, called *Chi*, flows along fourteen channels (meridians) throughout the body. Along each meridian are numerous acupuncture points, and by inserting special needles to stimulate these points, the flow of *Chi* is altered.

Acupuncture has been tried in the West for pain relief and for many disorders. Does it work for epilepsy? I was curious about it, and when some of my patients whose seizures were very resistant to drugs asked whether acupuncture would help them, I arranged for a small trial to check it out. All of them reported that acupuncture made them feel better. Unfortunately, their seizure diaries showed that all of them still had seizures just as frequently. So if you are happy to look on acupuncture as a kind of tonic, something to improve your general well-being but that probably will not have much effect on your seizures, go for it.

Meditation

There are many meditation techniques, but all of them have the same aim, which is to still the mind by emptying it of thoughts and anxieties. Many people manage to ward off migraine, for example, by meditating when they feel an attack coming on. Although there have been no studies to prove conclusively that meditation reduces seizure frequency, it seems logical to expect that it might help to ward off seizures, as we know that many people find seizures are more likely to occur when they are in an anxious state or under stress.

If you want to learn to meditate you can either take a course or join a group from one of the organizations that teach a meditation technique. Or you can practise this do-it-yourself mantra meditation method. Choose as your mantra a neutral word or sound which has no emotional overtones for you; it does not matter what it is.

1 Sit with your eyes closed and your back straight in a quiet room on an upright (but comfortable) chair.
2 Repeat your mantra silently to yourself, focusing all your attention on it. When thoughts come into your mind (which they will) do not actively try to banish them, but simply let them come and go, trying not to let yourself follow them.
3 Perform this exercise morning and evening each day if you can, and gradually you will find that it is easier to empty your mind of distracting thoughts. Practise for five or ten minutes at first, aiming to work up to 20 minutes meditation twice a day eventually.

Some people find it easier to empty their mind by focusing their attention on a visual image rather than by listening to a mantra. The principle is the same: to calm your mind by emptying it of thoughts and worries. You can also use a candle flame to help you. Look at the flame for a minute or so, then shut your eyes and keep your attention on the after-image which will appear in your mind. This after-image will change in colour and shape, but just watch it quite silently, all the time keeping your mind quiet.

Once you have become used to meditating, use it just as you would any other counter measure – whenever you feel a seizure is starting, or in any seizure-prone situation.

Yoga

Yoga is a system of Hindu philosophy which teaches mental and physical control by focusing attention. Like meditation or relaxation techniques, it can be practised in any situation where you feel you are likely to have a seizure. The two main forms of yoga practised in the West are hatha yoga, in which the practitioner adopts a series of physical poses, and prana yoga, in which attention is focused first on the 'in' breath and then on the 'out' breath. A yoga class will also teach relaxation techniques. Choose your teacher carefully, however: hatha yoga can create health problems if it is not taught properly or is practised by someone in poor health.

chapter six

Controlling Your Own Seizures

*M*arion's first seizure occurred when she was 14. She was at school, and had just been enjoying a quiet smoke with a few friends in a secluded corner of the playground, which was unfortunately not quite secluded enough. A sharp-eyed maths mistress with a keen sense of smell spotted a curl of smoke. As she was marching them off to see the Headmaster, Marion saved the day (or so her friends described it later) by having a seizure right there in the middle of the playground.

Marion never smoked again, because she always had a feeling that the cigarette must have somehow triggered her seizure. But she did continue to have seizures, and unfortunately they proved difficult to control. Eventually, some years later, she was referred to me. I questioned her closely about what happened when she had a seizure. When Marion thought about this she discovered that there was a pattern, though she had never realized it. She had had a seizure that morning, just after her husband had drawn her attention to the fact that he had no clean shirts. She had had a seizure a few days ago at work, soon after she had mislaid an important document. She remembered a seizure she'd had some weeks back, when she had just bought a dress which cost approximately twice what she had intended to spend. And it was then that she remembered *her first seizure of all. That fitted the pattern too; it wasn't the cigarette that had triggered the seizure, it was simply a strong feeling of guilt.*

'So now what you have to do,' I said to her, 'is to find some way to stop feeling guilty. Whenever you feel the guilt creeping on, why not try asking yourself: "How much is this going to matter in 20 years' time?" And if the answer's, "Not at all," then why feel guilty about it?'

When Marion tried this technique she found that she did indeed have fewer seizures. In fact, she described her new guilt-free attitude to life as the best anticonvulsant she had ever been prescribed!

Treatment with drugs is the best way to control seizures for nearly everyone. But it is not the only way. A new and less conventional approach to seizure control is called behavioural treatment, and it is based on the observation that by altering your behaviour you can often alter the pattern of your seizures.

Learning about your seizures

Seizures do not always occur at random. They are intimately related to how you feel, what you are doing, and what you are thinking. Most people with epilepsy will tell you that there are situations in which seizures are likely to occur, and others in which they seem to get fewer seizures, or even to be seizure free. You may have learnt that you tend to have seizures if you do not get enough sleep, for example, or if you miss meals so that your blood sugar level is low. For some people, flickering lights often cause seizures (see *Photosensitive Epilepsy*, pp.124–6).

Many people have fewer seizures on holiday, or when their interest is held, as at the theatre. Others find that a peaceful, low-key life style, without too much excitement or novelty, helps keep them seizure free. One study of adolescents found (perhaps not surprisingly) that they were far more likely to have a seizure if they were helping around the home than if they were relaxing by the fire.

THOUGHTS AND SEIZURES

Stress and other emotions are not the only factors which seem to influence the generation of seizures. If you have complex partial seizures (see p.12) activity in the nerve cells around the damaged area of brain from which seizures arise may be sufficient to start a seizure. Some seizures can sometimes be triggered by a particular mental process: doing mental arithmetic, for example. If seizures start in the part of the brain that is involved in mathematical calculations, for example, then adding or subtracting figures may precipitate a seizure. Some people find they have a seizure when they think sad thoughts, or feel angry or even (as in Marion's case, quoted above) when they feel guilty. In some people a seizure may be triggered when they are imagining three-dimensional objects: thinking about diagrams or planning moves in a chess game. One man, a motor mechanic, reported that he often had a seizure when he was tightening a nut in an inaccessible part of an engine; because he could not actually see the nut, he had to visualize what he was doing as he did it.

People who have seizures will often tell you that they have discovered they can stop a seizure, or prevent it spreading, by some mental or physical trick they have discovered, usually by accident or trial and error. When patients in an epilepsy out-patient clinic were asked about whether they had some mental strategy which helped inhibit their seizures, more than a third said that they had. They were not always successful, but most found that they could at least reduce the number of seizures they had.

The essence of many of these methods is distraction – turning your attention right away from the area of the body in which the seizure starts. It may help just to start thinking about something else, or to stop whatever it is you are doing and do something different. Often some quite simple trick helps to focus your attention elsewhere; some people like to have an elastic band around their wrist which they can tweak when they are aware that a seizure is beginning. Twisting a ring on your finger or an ear-ring in your ear for a few minutes can have the same effect. If your seizures usually start with the movement of a particular limb, holding the limb still to prevent movement may inhibit the seizure. Relaxation is also very successful for many people, and a relaxation method you can teach yourself is described above on pp.81–5.

Not everyone has the same trigger-factors. But if you can work out which your personal trigger-factors are, then you may be able to develop strategies to avoid them or reduce their frequency by altering your behaviour.

Some of the self-help methods described in this chapter depend on being able to recognize the warning or aura which indicates that a seizure may be going to occur. These methods will not work for you if you have generalized seizures which come out of the blue, with no warning or aura. But whatever kind of seizures you have, looking at them in the context of your whole life, and learning to modify your life style and avoid situations which you know are likely to precipitate a seizure will be helpful.

Looking for links

If you want to try to learn to control your own seizures, the first step is to learn to identify the things that are most likely to precipitate them. It will help you to keep a 'seizure diary' for at least a few months; and it will also help your doctor to have a record of your seizures and of what seems to trigger them off.

Best of all is to try the 'ABC' programme, which is the driving force of any programme of behavioural treatment carried out in hospital.

ABC CHARTS

An ABC chart is a detailed record of every seizure, describing what happens immediately before the seizure (A = Antecedents); behaviour (B) during the seizure; and what the consequences (C) of the seizure are for you. All you will need is a special A4 notebook to write your account in – and some honest observation. As well as this, mark every seizure you have on a wall chart or calendar which shows you the years at a glance. If your behavioural programme works, you should be able to watch your seizure frequency fall.

Antecedents
The antecedents of a seizure are particularly important. Try to remember exactly what was happening just before the seizure started. It will help if you ask yourself these questions:

- What were you doing just before the seizure/at seizure onset?
- How did you feel just before the seizure/at seizure onset?
- What were you thinking just before the seizure/at seizure onset?

It is important to be as precise as possible when you are answering these questions. If you can recognize and record your emotions it may help you identify those that may give rise to a seizure. Supposing, for example, that you had been looking at photographs of a previous summer holiday. It is not enough simply to say, 'I was looking through an old photograph album.' A more precise answer might have been: 'I was looking at a picture of Bob and me holding hands. I was feeling a bit sad.' If you can recall just what you were thinking at the moment the seizure started, so much the better: 'I was feeling jealous because Bob's got a new girlfriend now.' By analysing what happened in this way, you may be able to pinpoint the thoughts or feelings that led directly to the seizure.

Behaviour

You need to note down in as much detail as possible how your behaviour changed at the onset of the seizure. This will be important when you are trying to find a counter measure to inhibit your seizures (see below). For example, the first change in behaviour might have been the movement of a limb, or a thought or a feeling, or perhaps a strange feeling like butterflies in the pit of your stomach which moved up into the chest. To fill in the details you may have to ask someone who was with you at the time. List everything you can.

If you are worried about your behaviour during a seizure – the fact that you may have been incontinent for example – do discuss this with your doctor or someone close to you. Sometimes video monitoring of a seizure (see p.88) can reassure you that whatever aspect of your behaviour in a seizure worries you is not so terrible after all.

Consequences

Consequences are important. Try to note down in detail not only what happened immediately after the seizure, but how it may have changed the situation for you, and also how you felt. People quite often feel despondent, even guilty, about having had another seizure, and, again, if your doctor knows how you feel he can help you tackle these feelings.

If, as a parent, you are trying to keep an ABC chart for a child who has seizures, you may find that consequences are especially significant. The child who has a seizure in class, for example, and is taken out of class and given milk and biscuits by a sympathetic teacher, is being given a strong message – seizures are likely to be rewarded! It is far better to encourage the child to return to the classroom as soon as they have recovered, and to withold the milk and biscuits. But adults too are sometimes 'rewarded' by a seizure. If you discover from your chart that you regularly have a seizure after an argument with a partner for example, and always find that he or she is remorseful and attentive towards you afterwards, you could learn something useful!

Interpreting your charts
Once you start looking for links, it is very likely that you will be able to find some sort of relationship between the likelihood of a seizure occurring and your physiological state: whether you were particularly tired or hungry, for example, your emotions, what you were doing, or what was going on in your life with family and friends.

Finding a counter measure

The aim of the ABC chart is to help you see the behaviour that is most likely to precipitate a seizure and enable you or your doctor to work out appropriate counter measures to help you control your seizures.

A counter measure is a piece of behaviour which you use either to inhibit the seizure completely, or at least to stop its spread. The counter measure is carried out either when you are in a situation in which you know a seizure is likely to occur, or at the beginning of a seizure.

Counter measures are often strategies which lead either to an increase or decrease in arousal or alertness. The A of your ABC chart may, for example, show that you are more likely to have seizures when you are aroused – excited or tense. In this case a relaxation technique would be a good counter measure (see p.81).

You would use an alerting strategy if you found that you were most likely to get a seizure when you were day-dreaming or in a very boring situation. One patient with complex partial seizures found he could often abort a seizure just by saying 'No' to himself, or attending to something different at the onset of the aura. Another found hitting his arm would sometimes abort a seizure. Arousing yourself by walking about, pinching yourself, or distracting yourself either in seizure-prone situations or at seizure onset, is often effective. Some of the alternative methods of seizure control discussed in the last chapter, for example aromatherapy and relaxation techniques, probably work at least partly because they help you to change your level of arousal quickly when you feel a seizure beginning.

Many patients, particularly if they have complex partial seizures, have a seizure onset related to negative emotions such as anxiety or unhappiness. Here the counter measure would be designed either to help you avoid such thoughts, or to distract attention from them. Some people find that sniffing at a bottle of old-fashioned smelling salts, or indeed any substance with a powerful smell, can distract attention from feelings of anxiety and inhibit a seizure. An elastic band around the wrist, twanged at seizure onset, has the same effect. (This can be a way of arousing or alerting yourself, too).

Learning to avoid feelings such as unhappiness or guilt that trigger a seizure is obviously more difficult than simply distracting your attention from them. But once you recognize the part these feelings play, you can at least make an attempt to adjust your life so that you experience them less often.

Sometimes counter measures can be very specific. For example, if a seizure usually starts with the same movement, such as flexing an arm, it can often be stopped if you deliberately make an opposing movement – in this case, straightening the arm.

Whatever counter measure you use, enter all your seizures on your annual plan chart so that you can see how successful the counter measure is at reducing your seizure frequency.

Making seizures happen

There is, of course, another side to this coin. If so many people have the ability to stop a seizure, it is not surprising that quite a lot find that they can make a seizure happen deliberately without too much difficulty. Many people know that they can bring on their own seizures by a direct act of will, by thinking or behaving in a certain way. Probably many more do the very same thing without realizing that they are doing so. If seizures start with a movement such as flexing a limb or turning the head, then mimicking the movement while mentally willing a seizure to occur may actually precipitate one. In one survey of people attending an epilepsy clinic about a quarter of the interviewees said they could generate a seizure at will. However, this figure is probably an over-estimate: a study of Swedish children with epilepsy found that 16 per cent could make themselves have a seizure if they tried. But, more importantly, *all* of these children said that they knew the circumstances in which they were likely to have a seizure.

> *Lucy's father died when she was 14. At the time she was intensely miserable, and used to lie on her bed every evening crying. Lucy had epilepsy, and she found that often when she was feeling very sad she would have a seizure. She came to welcome these seizures because they meant that for a short time at least she was unconscious and therefore free of her misery.*
>
> *Eventually Lucy got over her father's death. For several years her seizures were well controlled. Then, seemingly out of the blue, one evening she started having recurrent seizures and was taken to hospital as an emergency. Afterwards, when questioned closely by her doctor, Lucy admitted that she had recently broken up with her boyfriend. The day of her hospital admission she had been lying on her bed, feeling very sad, just as she had when her father died. She had had a seizure, and felt that in the seizure she was able to escape from her*

sadness. Coming out of the seizure she was overwhelmed by misery once again and had allowed the sad feelings to sweep over her, knowing that it would result in another seizure . . . and another . . . and another.

People who have discovered that emotional mental states such as sadness or resentment can cause seizures, for example, can often ensure that they have a seizure by deliberately thinking about things that they know make them feel sad or resentful. It is not unheard of for children to use this kind of ploy when a parent is angry with them.

Some people find that deliberately keeping their mind blank can precipitate a seizure. You may discover quite by accident what particular movement or mental activity always seems to start a seizure off, or that you can will a seizure by manipulating your attention or thinking certain thoughts. It is very common, for instance, for people to have seizures when they are thinking or talking about seizures.

There is thus a very fine line between deliberately inducing a seizure and allowing yourself the luxury of a mental state or a behaviour that you know is likely to induce one.

It would be nice to be able to say that there is a good chance you may be able to control your epilepsy completely by using behavioural methods. Unfortunately, this is not very likely. These self-help methods are not meant to replace drugs, and you certainly should not stop taking your drugs if you practise them. But they are a useful addition to more conventional treatment.

A complete treatment of epilepsy does not involve just taking drugs. It means learning how your feelings, thinking and behaviour can all be used in the control of your seizures. You will not then be nearly so much at the mercy of your epilepsy. You will be able to gain some mastery over your seizures instead of letting them control you and dominate your life.

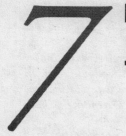

*I*t was the day of the end of term Christmas concert, and Carol, aged 15, was waiting in the wings, just about to go on and play her piano solo. Her family, sitting in the front row, were excited because her young brother was just out of hospital after lengthy treatment for a childhood illness. Carol's parents had had a difficult four years during their son's illness, the low point of which came when Carol's mother had a confrontation with the specialist over diagnosis. She had determinedly and single-mindedly sought a second opinion which led to successful treatment.

As she made her way onto the platform, Marian tripped and fell heavily on her arm. She managed her performance but was clearly in pain. That evening at home she looked flushed and feverish. She stayed in bed for the next two days and when she got up she felt dizzy, and her injured arm was weak. Matters didn't improve and by the end of the week she could hardly use her arm and her GP referred her to a specialist. The specialist (a neurologist) told her that there was nothing wrong with the arm except some minor bruising. But her mother was certain it was more than this and insisted that Carol should be admitted to hospital for investigation.

The specialist finally agreed to take Carol into hospital. On the neurological ward were several patients with severe epilepsy, and during her first day there Carol saw several grand mal seizures. That evening she had her first 'seizure'. This consisted *of thrashing side-to-side movements of her head which went on for some twenty minutes. The houseman diagnosed epilepsy and treated her with intravenous diazepam and informed her parents of the diagnosis.*

Every evening she was in hospital Carol had a similar attack, but meanwhile all tests and investigations, even an EEG, had proved normal. Eventually Carol was told that she didn't have epilepsy at all, but that she was 'pretending' to have these attacks. She was discharged and sent home.

Back in the bosom of her family Carol, predictably, had another attack that evening which lasted for four hours. Her distraught father rang the hospital and was told she was play-acting. This situation continued for the next two weeks, with Carol having attacks every night. The local neurologist was again persuaded to see her, said he had nothing to offer, and that Carol should see a psychiatrist. But Carol's mother, sensitized by her son's experience and clinging to the house-man's original diagnosis of epilepsy, refused to accept a psychological cause and sought second (and third, and fourth) opinions elsewhere. She was finally referred to a specialist unit, with the diagnosis of 'unusual epileptic seizures'.

For the first week on the unit Carol would have an attack every night, after which she became exhausted and fell asleep. Video monitoring of the attacks showed that they were quite unchar-acteristic of any form of epileptic seizure. If she was spoken to during an attack she would sometimes reply. Her attacks were so clearly *not* epileptic in nature that it was not even necessary to have the additional evidence of a normal EEG during an attack to clinch the diagnosis.

A small number of people who are at first diagnosed as having epilepsy are eventually found to have non-epileptic seizures. Their seizures can look very much like epileptic seizures, and indeed they are easily mistaken for epilepsy by the doctors who examine them, most of whom may not have had special training in epilepsy. But when they are given an electroencephalogram during an attack, it does not show the characteristic patterns of a true epileptic seizure.

Non-epileptic seizures usually serve some purpose. They are often an expression of the person's emotional needs, and play a role in helping them cope with difficulties in their emotional life. It has been found that people who have been sexually abused as children quite often develop non-epileptic seizures (though of course this does not mean that everyone who has non-epileptic seizures has been sexually abused, or that everyone who has been sexually abused has non-epileptic seizures).

Carol herself was a teenager with a poor self-image and almost complete lack of self-confidence. She was finding the transition from childhood to adulthood hard and needed emotional support from her family, particularly her mother, which she was not getting. Eventually Carol was able to talk to her doctor about her deep unhappiness about her relationship with her parents, particularly with her mother. She had seen how her brother's illness had occupied her mother's complete attention over the last four years. Wanting her mother's love and support, she felt, with some reason, that only 'proper' illnesses interested her mother. Was it surprising that she felt the only way she could get the same degree of attention was by developing a 'proper' illness herself?

Confusion about diagnosis

Sometimes, as in Carol's case, the diagnosis of non-epileptic seizures is easily made. But often diagnosis is not so easy, and occasionally it presents a real problem for both the doctor and the patient, who may be given anticonvulsants unnecessarily over many years.

Someone who has non-epileptic seizures usually has a model on which to base them. Sometimes someone else in the family has epilepsy, or the person has had some similar experience such as a faint. In Carol's case she had had expert, though unintentional, tutoring by the people on her ward who experienced genuine seizures.

A few people have both non-epileptic seizures and epileptic seizures. It is important that both should be diagnosed because both need to be treated, and treatment is different.

Diagnosis of non-epileptic seizures is particularly difficult in people who have both epilepsy and non-epileptic seizures, and who therefore have a very good model of epilepsy on which to build their non-epileptic attacks. Indeed, the person experiencing both kinds of attacks often finds it difficult to distinguish between the two for him or herself. They will usually say, for example, that their non-epileptic attacks seem to come out of the blue just like real epilepsy. It does not seem to them that they are feigning attacks. Nevertheless, these non-epileptic attacks can nearly always be distinguished from an epileptic seizure.

When someone who has epilepsy also develops non-epileptic seizures there is a problem in treatment as well as diagnosis. Even if the frequency of the person's epileptic seizures is actually being reduced, their doctor may not realize that this is the case because the person continues to have non-epileptic seizures. They may be given even higher doses of anticonvulsant drugs which they do not need.

Why should someone who has genuine epilepsy develop non-epileptic seizures too? Quite often the real epileptic seizures have been more or less brought under control, but the patient still 'needs' their seizures, perhaps for the attention they bring, or because they allow him or her to remain dependent. It may take time for someone to learn to do without their seizures.

Not surprisingly, then, the patient with non-epileptic seizures is often given different diagnoses. Some doctors diagnose epilepsy, others non-epileptic seizures. No wonder the patients themselves are often confused about what they do have, or that they often reject medical help if the advice they are given is conflicting. Even more important, a prolonged non-epileptic seizure may be mistaken for *status epilepticus* (see p.22) and the patient rushed to the nearest intensive care unit and given treatment which is entirely appropriate for someone who *is* in *status epilepticus*, but highly dangerous for anyone else. So although non-epileptic seizures are not dangerous in themselves, they should never be taken lightly.

Treating non-epileptic seizures

At present there is no real consensus amongst doctors about the most effective way to treat someone who has non-epileptic seizures. Sometimes (though not usually in specialist epilepsy units) a very confrontational approach is used: the 'snap out of it and stop trying to pull the wool over our eyes' school of treatment. This does not work because it blames the person for something which is not their fault and ignores the very important fact that *all* seizures, whether they are organic or emotional, have a cause. Above all, it does not take into account that these non-epileptic seizures can be just as disabling and disruptive for the patient as a 'real' seizure.

Treatment of non-epileptic seizures needs to be carried out in a specialist unit. The first step is to start investigating the seizures. The more thorough the investigation, the less easy it will be for the patient rationally to reject the suggestion that their seizures are not due to epilepsy.

At the same time the patient will be reassured that although the attacks are not epileptic but emotional, they are nonetheless real, and are due to a build-up of tension and emotion. They are also told that non-epileptic seizures need to be treated just as do epileptic ones. But the best news as far as the patient is concerned is that the seizures are more easily cured and the patient can learn to control their own attacks.

Each patient is given a key nurse to whom they can talk at any time. The relationship between the patient and the nursing and medical staff is crucial, because it is only when trust has built up between them that the patient will feel able to talk freely about the tensions in their life and the difficulties they are having, at work or at home.

RECOGNIZING TRIGGER SITUATIONS

The next step is for the patient to be shown how to analyse the situations in which they have attacks, and to recognize that there may sometimes be emotional triggers for their attacks. This is done in very much the same way that people who have epileptic seizures are taught to recognize situations which may trigger a seizure (see p.17).

They will be taught to analyse exactly what is happening to them just before an attack starts, in particular asking themselves:

- What were they doing just before the attack?
- How did they feel just before the attack?
- What were they thinking just before the attack?

If they can recognize and record their emotions very precisely, they may be able to identify the thoughts that make them have an attack. Maybe they were feeling very tense; perhaps someone had been angry with them or spoken sharply to them and their feelings were hurt; or maybe some memory had come into their mind that was too painful to think about.

The patient is asked to think about the consequences of the attack too, and to note down in as much detail as possible not only what happened immediately after the attack, but how it may have altered the situation for them, and how they felt. If they were very tense beforehand, for example, did they feel much better after the attack? If they had been feeling very lonely or ignored beforehand, were people comforting them or paying them attention afterwards?

Usually, if they manage this sort of analysis honestly, most people can find some sort of connection between the likelihood of an attack occurring and their feelings, what is going on in their life or their relationships with other people.

BEHAVIOURAL PROGRAMMES

The patient is then given a behavioural treatment programme similar to that described on p.109. They will be taught to recognize situations in which they are likely to have an attack, but to try to *talk* about how they feel instead of allowing their feelings to precipitate an attack. They will be taught a method of relaxation (see pp.81–5), and shown how to use relaxation whenever they feel they might have an attack. They are encouraged to admit that their attacks are emotional and not epileptic. And they are helped to talk about their problems and anxieties rather than their seizures.

Finally, they have to be helped to come to terms with an absence of seizures and decide how they are going to run their life seizure free. The family is always involved in this phase of treatment, for they too will have to decide how they are going to respond to the patient's absence of seizures.

The success of the treatment depends a great deal on how much the person still needs their seizures. The problems that created the need for seizures do not just disappear once the attacks stop, and they still somehow have to be resolved. The sufferer has to learn how to get his or her emotional needs met more straightforwardly, and the family have to be taught how to offer the support the patient needs. If these strategies can not be worked out, non-epileptic seizures are a problem that can persist.

Non-Epileptic Seizures: A Diagnosis Checklist

- Do the seizures fail to respond to drugs?
- Is consciousness maintained during a seizure?
- Does the person seldom hurt themselves badly during a violent seizure?
- Do they feel better after a seizure rather than worse?
- Do their seizures last for a very long time?
- Do their seizures involve very complex bodily movements, thrashing about or waving of limbs?

If the answers to all these questions are **yes** then it is **possible** that seizures are emotional and not epileptic in origin. At any rate, this is a possibility that the doctor will want to consider.

8

Living with Epilepsy

*O*ne wet and windy afternoon Sue Usiskin was passing her local building society when she recognized the first signs of one of her usual seizures. Wasting no time she entered, beckoning for help as she crumpled to the floor.

'The seizure gained momentum. I felt very conspicuous as, apart from myself, the place was empty. The staff stayed exactly where they were behind the counter. None of them came to my aid as I shook and groaned.

'Eventually the seizure subsided and I lay wondering how I might get one of the staff to ring my husband at his office nearby. As soon as I was able, I crawled across the floor to the counter, clutching my epilepsy card. I indicated my husband's work number on it and fortunately he appeared in minutes. The manager, who was still behind the counter, explained that he thought I was the diversion for a robbery and had he come to my aid there would have been a chance for an accomplice to get behind the counter.' (From *Women and Epilepsy*, John Wiley and Sons 1991).

The problem with fits is that they are unpredictable. They can disrupt your daily routine, your education, your social life and your work. Often they provoke anxiety in others which can alter their relationship with you in subtle ways. And very occasionally, your seizures may have catastrophic consequences.

111

People who have epilepsy have always suffered as much from other peoples' attitudes towards them and their condition as from the disease itself. Someone who has epilepsy may no longer be considered mad or possessed by the devil, but they are still often regarded, at the very least, as different and liable to occasional bouts of strange behaviour which may embarrass or distress the onlooker who does not understand them and does not know how to cope with them. The epilepsy sufferer may have to contend with other people's belief that they are somehow second-class citizens, unable to live a normal life. It is often assumed that epilepsy is some form of mental handicap or that it causes a deterioration of personality, or even that it can be caught, like flu.

Sue Usiskin, herself an epilepsy counsellor whose experience is quoted above, says she always makes a point of going back to see people where she has had a seizure. If they have been helpful they usually appreciate seeing her well and having the chance to ask her questions about the condition. To those who have not been so helpful she offers some basic education about epilepsy in the form of a leaflet giving information about first aid for fits.

Shaping other people's attitudes

The person who has epilepsy is someone who happens to have an occasional fit; between seizures he or she is as normal and capable as the person who happens to have an occasional cold. Such people do not need or want sympathy or special treatment. There are endless examples of famous people throughout history whose epilepsy clearly proved to be no barrier to the achievement of fame and even fortune. Julius Caesar, Alexander the Great and Alfred the Great were all said to have had epilepsy. The writers Jane Austen and Dostoevsky had epilepsy and so did the poet Byron. Tony Greig had epilepsy and captained the English cricket team.

In almost every case, other people's attitudes towards your epilepsy will reflect your own. If you regard it as a minor nuisance – something you have to live with but that need not affect your capacity for life or make you different or in need of sympathy or special treatment – your friends, colleagues and the people you meet in your everyday life will adopt this view too.

However, it is sensible to warn friends and work colleagues what they should do if you have a seizure (see p.133). If you have generalized tonic clonic seizures the important point to make is that, however horrifying it looks to them, it is not painful or distressing for you, because you are not in any real sense 'there' while it is happening.

Taking control of your life

Sam was 22 years old and pleased with life. He'd had tonic clonic, grand mal seizures since he was 15, but these were well controlled. He had just got a job he really enjoyed as a management trainee in a local supermarket, and (even more important for Sam) had left home and for the first time was living in a flat on his own. Then things started to go wrong. His seizure frequency started to increase: five mornings during his first couple of months at work he had a seizure soon after he arrived at the supermarket. His mother said she had known this would happen. She said that Sam should come to live at home again. 'No way', was Sam's reply.

When Sam came to see me I asked him about the job. Was he finding it more difficult than he'd expected? Were his employers sympathetic? But it soon seemed clear that it wasn't stress that was causing the increase in seizures – Sam was very happy at work, found the job easy, liked the people he worked with and hadn't met with anything but support and encouragement even when he had seizures.

'Well then,' I said, 'tell me about your day.'

'That's easy,' Sam replied.

He got up around 7.55, was out of the house by 8.15 to

catch the 8.30 train and was at work by 8.55. After work he'd come home, have supper, listen to some music and do some studying, and be in bed by midnight. I asked him if he thought that was a sensible routine, and he said yes, very. He knew it was important for him to get enough sleep, and that way he got his eight hours; he'd even tried getting up at 8.15 but found he missed his train more often than not, so stuck to 7.55.

It was obvious that on that timetable something had to go, and I had a strong suspicion I knew what it was.

'What about breakfast?' I asked Sam. He looked very defensive. He didn't feel like eating first thing in the morning and one of the problems about living at home had been his mother's determination to force a good breakfast down him every morning. Now he was on his own he'd rather have 20 minutes extra in bed, thank you very much.

However, Sam agreed to try the treatment I recommended, and I'm pleased to report that it worked like a dream. Sam's the only patient I've been able to cure simply by prescribing a bowl of cornflakes and two pieces of toast and marmalade taken after waking, before work, every morning.

Many people report that they have seizures when they are hungry. It is not really clear why this happens. Certainly a very low blood sugar level can cause a seizure, as sometimes happens when someone who has diabetes has not eaten properly or takes too much insulin, but blood sugar seldom falls this low in someone who does not suffer from diabetes, even when they are hungry. However, even if we do not properly understand why, it still seems that having a good breakfast and eating regular meals during the day help many people keep the frequency of their seizures low.

It is easy to become dependent when you have epilepsy, and let other people try to control your life. Things do not have to be like that. But if you want to take control of your own life, you must take control of the factors which affect your seizures.

First, you need a good doctor: someone who is up to date and will put you on to the best drugs, and will listen to what you have to say. When you have found him or her, see them often, have frequent blood tests, and follow their advice.

Second, try to harmonize your life, so that you eliminate, or at least modify, those factors which tend to precipitate your seizures.

Eating sensibly is a beginning. Tiredness is another factor which is known very often to increase the frequency of seizures, and it too is more or less under your control. Do not get overtired or have too many late nights.

There is plenty of evidence that stress can precipitate seizures. But stress can be a subtle and complex problem. Some people give themselves seizures by winding themselves up to a high stress level and then relaxing again. For others stress or even intense excitement may in itself cause seizures. Some people tend to have seizures when they become very stressed and then relax again. You have to find out what sort of person you are, and what particular pattern of stress and relaxation affects you. Only then can you see how to modify your life style and change the pattern.

Fourteen-year-old Simon loved making models. He would sit for two hours or more at a time, oblivious to everything around him, concentrating only on each tiny plastic part as he carefully manoeuvred it into its correct place.

When he had finished he would fling himself into an armchair, lean back and say, 'Phew!' That was when he was most likely to have a seizure. He had another seizure-prone time too, during one of his favourite times of day – that pleasant half hour on a weekend morning when he would wake and lie there lazily, knowing he didn't have to get up and go to school.

Simon's doctor pointed out to him that his seizures seemed much less frequent when he was alert and aroused. He suggested that instead of relaxing straight away when he'd finished his model building, Simon should put the model away, and then go for a walk round the house for five or ten minutes before sitting down. When he tried this, Simon found that he did indeed have fewer seizures. His doctor also suggested that he should arouse himself a bit more quickly on weekend mornings – get up and do something rather than lie in bed. This wasn't a popular suggestion, but it did stop Simon's early morning weekend seizures.

Happiness – a good anticonvulsant

You may also have noticed that you are more likely to have a seizure if you are in a particular mental state. Some people find that getting very angry, or feeling guilty or ashamed, tends to bring on a seizure. Dealing with this kind of seizure precipitant requires a good deal of mental discipline, but it can be done.

The link between seizures and emotions is a long and well-established one. As long ago as 1901, when really very little was known about epilepsy, Dr William Gower, one of the first physicians to specialize in the condition, described the part he believed emotion played in the generation of seizures:

> 'Of all the immediate causes of epilepsy the most potent are psychical – fright, excitement, anxiety . . . of the three forms of emotion, fright takes the first place . . . One case was that of a soldier who had his first fit a few hours after being terrified, while on sentry duty at night, by the unexpected appearance of some white goats on the top of the adjacent wall of a cemetery which he mistook for emissaries from the graves.'

Fright probably does not rank as a number one precipitant of seizures for as many people nowadays but Dr Gower's general principle is just as valid today. Over one third of people with epilepsy describe an emotional precipitant: excitement, anger, tension and anxiety seem to be the most common.

Even in animals this also seems to be the case. It has been shown, for example, that anxiety and stress can increase epileptic spiking in the EEG of monkeys, and induce seizures. A group of monkeys will establish a 'pecking order' or dominance hierarchy, and it has been found that epileptic monkeys low in the dominance hierarchy had a larger number of spikes and more seizures when they were exposed to monkeys higher up the hierarchy.

Finally, be happy. Happiness seems to be one of the most effective anticonvulsants. It has been noticed that children with epilepsy tend to have fewer fits when they are enjoying themselves. Keeping your relationships with other people tranquil will almost certainly help you keep down your seizures. Family rows often precipitate seizures, so keep on good terms with those around you if you can. And while it is both unrealistic and unnecessary to try to lead an entirely stress-free life, it is a good idea to notice whether you seem to be more seizure-prone when you are het up or under stress. If so, it will help to learn a method of relaxation which you can practise when you feel the tension building up.

You can not be happy to order, but most of us have at least some control over our own moods. When we feel slightly depressed, it is easy to let ourselves deliberately slide further down into despondency by thinking even more miserable thoughts. There are people who seem almost to cultivate an air of perpetual gloom, while others manage to keep reasonably cheerful most of the time. Being happy is probably a combination of personality and sheer effort, but anyone can make the effort. It is especially important to work at your personal relationships and keep them in good order, because most of us are dependent on our close relationships for a good deal of our happiness.

Diet and epilepsy

There is very little evidence that modifying your diet can affect the number or severity of your seizures. However, some people do notice that certain foods seem to precipitate attacks (milk seems to do it for some people, chocolate or coffee for others). So it is worth looking at your diet to see whether seizures do tend to occur more often after some particular food or drink. If you think they do, test out your theory! Give up the food for a month and mark on your seizure chart the date that you gave it up. At the end of one month see if you have had fewer seizures than in the previous month. Then reintroduce the food into your diet, marking your chart with the date you started eating it again. After another month, check the number of seizures you have had. If your seizure frequency has gone up again, it might be worth eliminating that particular food for good. Sometimes this dietary modification works for an individual, even if we know of no scientific reason why it should.

EVENING PRIMROSE OIL

Evening primrose oil is a popular remedy, widely used to relieve symptoms in a huge variety of conditions, including eczema, premenstrual syndrome, rheumatoid arthritis and asthma. Although it is generally a very safe treatment, evening primrose oil should not be taken if you have, or have ever had, epilepsy, or if you have a strong family history of epilepsy. Evening primrose oil actually has the potential to precipitate symptoms of un-diagnosed temporal lobe epilepsy.

THE KETOGENIC DIET

Fasting has long been known to be one way of reducing seizure frequency. What happens in fasting conditions is that body fat is broken down to produce energy. No one knows why this should

118

reduce seizure frequency in people with epilepsy, but there is no doubt that in some it does. One theory is that the breakdown of fats on a large scale makes the body more acidic, and from experience it has been found that this acidity acts as an anti-convulsant.

The ketogenic diet is a diet which contains a very large proportion of saturated fat (animal fats and some vegetable oils), and a drastically reduced proportion of protein and carbohydrate, so that about 90 per cent of the body's daily energy requirements come from fat. (In a normal, healthy Western diet fat provides 30–35 per cent of the daily energy needs.) So, just as happens in fasting conditions, the massive breakdown of fats makes the body more acidic, and this is probably why the diet tends to reduce seizure frequency.

There is nothing new about the ketogenic diet. In fact it is one of the oldest treatments for epilepsy. The real problem with the diet is that it is both extraordinarily nasty and very difficult to prepare. Very few adults ever tolerate it for long, though it is occasionally given to children as a last resort. But since the first really effective anticonvulsant drug, phenytoin, appeared on the market the diet has largely fallen into disuse, and nobody has much regretted its passing.

So why, now in the 1990s, has the ketogenic diet suddenly re-emerged, like Frankenstein, from what most people would consider a timely grave? The answer to this question provides a very good example of medication by media.

The diet's new-found popularity is due largely to an American film producer whose child has epilepsy. Despite numerous visits to eminent neurologists who tried every possible drug, the child's seizures proved almost impossible to control. In desperation the father researched epilepsy treatments in the local library and came across the ketogenic diet, which no one had suggested to him.

He introduced his child to the diet and was very fortunate in that the child's epilepsy improved. He then made a video film describing the way the diet had miraculously transformed his child's life (and, rather unfairly, how all the doctors he had seen had failed to help). The film was seen widely on television. A

119

spate of articles in the popular press followed, and the ketogenic diet is now the rage in the United States; there are also signs that parents in many other parts of the world are starting to ask why this miracle treatment has not been prescribed for their children.

How effective the diet really is, is still a matter of medical debate. The enthusiasts (and they include some very eminent doctors) say as many as half the children who try it achieve a 50 per cent reduction in seizures. Those who are less enthusiastic, though equally reputable, quote figures of around 5 per cent or less. No one doubts that it works for some children, or that when it does fail it is often because it is difficult to apply properly, and heartily disliked by the child.

There are also questions about the long-term implications for a child's health which most parents (and doctors) will probably want answered before they embark on the ketogenic diet:

- **Will it make my child fat?**
  It should not do so if the diet is correctly balanced. The child's total daily calorie intake should not alter; what changes is the balance of foods. Only if the child eats more than they need to satisfy their daily energy requirements will they get fat.
- **Will it increase the chances of my child developing heart disease?**
  We are so conditioned to associate a high-fat diet with heart disease that it is difficult to believe that the ketogenic diet can be healthy. But in the short term at any rate there is no evidence that children who have been given the diet develop the fatty plaques in their blood vessels which are the cause of heart disease. However, for those few children who have a family history of high blood cholesterol (hyperlipoproteinaemia) the diet may be a real danger. Any child who starts the diet should be monitored carefully to check the levels of blood cholesterol.
- **Are there any other health problems associated with the diet?**
  A few children develop kidney stones on the diet, and it

may also have an effect on the immune system, though there is no evidence that this effect causes any significant problems in the short term.

If you are tempted to put your child on the ketogenic diet:

- Do not try it if your child's epilepsy is already well controlled by drugs.
- Do not try it unless you are able (and willing) to put a lot of time and effort into preparing your child's food.
- Do not try it unless you have a supportive medical team *including a trained dietician* to help you.
- Do not try it if there is any family history of high blood cholesterol.
- Think about how your child will feel. No child likes to be different. The child with epilepsy starts off with a built-in difference from other children which they have to learn to live with. It will not make them feel any better if they are debarred even from eating the same biscuits, buns, sweets, hamburgers, ice-creams – all the snacks and junk foods that their friends eat and which most children enjoy.

If you decide to try it:

- Learn all you can about food preparation. A skilled cook can make the diet much more acceptable – even, its supporters would say, quite appetizing.
- Encourage your child to become involved both in the choice of food and its preparation. They are much more likely to stick with it if they have some control over it.
- Be prepared for a difficult time at first as the child's body adjusts to the diet. To begin with the child may be irritable because their blood sugar is low, but after a week or two this should settle down.
- Listen to your child. If they really hate the diet, and many do, ask yourself if it is worth putting them through it for what may be only a small reduction in seizures.

121

- If, after three or four weeks, there has been no improvement in seizure control, give it up.

WATER LOAD

Some years ago a medical scare story was published in the press suggesting that a certain brand of lemonade had been found to cause seizures. The facts were rather different; the lemonade was entirely innocent. The seizures were not lemonade-induced but due to the fact that it had been a hot summer's day and the sufferer had drunk more than two litres of the stuff. He had given himself a huge 'water load' – too much liquid drunk too quickly, which is known sometimes to trigger a seizure.

When you are thirsty, do not drink huge amounts to quench your thirst. A glass of water is fine but if you drink, say, two or three pints all at one time you risk precipitating a seizure. There is no need to restrict your overall fluid intake, but try to drink little and often rather than allowing yourself to develop a real thirst that might make you want to drink very deeply.

Alcohol

Giles was a company director, successful, with a nice home, a family he loved and a good job. He had occasional grand mal seizures, and his doctor had advised him that he shouldn't drive and reminded him that it was a condition of his licence that he let the vehicle licensing department at Swansea know that he had been diagnosed as suffering from epilepsy. His doctor also warned him that he shouldn't drink alcohol.

Despite this, Giles insisted on driving. He was careful about drinking; although he drank occasionally he would nearly always stay within the legal limit, and he never drove after he'd been drinking. One evening he had a business dinner, and as he was getting a lift home, he drank about half a bottle of wine. The next morning as he was driving himself to work he had a seizure. His car struck an oncoming Rolls Royce, badly damaging it and injuring the owner's wife, who was a passenger. Unfortunately for Giles, an on-the-spot policeman saw what had happened, realized he had had a fit and reported him to the Licensing Authority. His insurance company was also informed; they wrote to his GP who confirmed that Giles did have seizures. The insurance company then refused to cover his claim, which was considerable as it included not only the Rolls but damages for injuries sustained by the passenger. Giles had to sell his house to meet the claim.

Of course, Giles should not have been driving at all, regardless of whether he had been drinking. In addition, he had not properly understood that it is withdrawal from alcohol that tends to trigger seizures, not the drinking itself.

You will have to drink with care while you are taking anticonvulsant drugs although you may not need to cut out alcohol altogether. There are several reasons for taking care with alcohol. It will react with your drugs and slow you down much more than you would expect. Alcohol causes what is known as 'liver enzyme induction'. It stimulates the liver to produce more enzymes which break it, and other drugs, down more rapidly so that it can be excreted. If you have one or two drinks a day regularly over a long period and then stop suddenly, the liver function returns to normal and your anticonvulsant drugs will not be broken down so fast. They also tend to accumulate in your blood. If you are taking phenytoin, the raised level of the drug may cause seizures; the raised levels of any other drugs you are taking may also have toxic effects. And, as discovered, if you have been drinking and then stop, alcohol withdrawal itself may precipitate a seizure.

If you have epilepsy, your best policy is not to drink at all. But if you find this impractical or impossible, do try to stick to these rules for safer drinking:

- Drink as little as possible and try not to develop a regular drinking habit, even if it is only a moderate one.
- Take 'shorts' or order half a pint of beer to avoid the water load that can sometimes precipitate a seizure.

Photosensitive epilepsy

Revolving disco lights are a notorious seizure trigger. But not everyone has the kind of epilepsy that is provoked by flickering lights. Those few people who do are said to have photosensitive epilepsy (PSE). In these people, watching television, flickering lights or even moving through shadows in bright sunlight may all trigger off a seizure. The rate of flicker seems to make a difference: 16–25 flashes per second is the rate most likely to precipitate a seizure. A rate of less than five flashes per second rarely induces seizures. The flickering must also be in the central part of your visual field to induce seizures; flickering that you see only out of the corner of your eye has little convulsant effect. However, going to the cinema very rarely provokes fits. About a third of people with photosensitive epilepsy are sensitive to pattern, especially chequerboard pattern.

Photosensitive epilepsy is mostly a disorder of children and adolescents. Although two per cent of people of all ages with seizures have PSE, in the age range 7–19 years the proportion rises to ten per cent. About one in four people lose their photosensitivity, usually before the age of 30.

Although television is the commonest trigger for seizures in people who have PSE, the fact that someone has a fit whilst watching TV does not necessarily mean that they have photo-sensitive epilepsy. In most Western countries people now watch so much television that inevitably some epilepsy sufferers will have a fit while sitting in front of the TV. Moreover, drowsiness is even more likely to induce fits than flickering lights, and a lot of TV-watching takes place in the evening, when people are drowsy anyway (or have TV-induced drowsiness). A diagnosis of photosensitive epilepsy can only be made from an EEG taken while the person is being stimulated by flashing lights.

Sodium valproate is the most successful drug for photosensitive epilepsy. However, it may not even be necessary for you to take anticonvulsant medication if you take these simple precautions to reduce your chances of having a seizure.

- Always watch TV from a distance of at least six feet (two metres).
- Watch a colour TV if possible, rather than a black and white one.
- You are less likely to get a seizure watching TV if the room is well lit. Put a small, lighted table lamp on top of the TV set.
- Use a remote control panel to change channels; do not go close to the set to adjust it or to switch channels.
- Avoid discos or any other situation in which you are likely to meet rapidly flashing lights or flickering patterns.
- If you find yourself in such a situation, cover ONE eye with a hand. Do this if you have to go near a TV set too. Do not close both your eyes to protect against flicker; this only seems to accentuate the effect and make you more likely to have a fit.
- Wear polarized sun glasses when you are out of doors on sunny days. They help to remove flickering reflections, especially beside the sea.

VDUs

In general VDUs cause no problems, because they do not have the same characteristics as TV sets. In very simple technical terms, most VDU monitors change the picture 70 times a second (70Hz), which is outside the photosensitive range of most people who have PSE, while in a standard TV monitor the picture changes only 25 times a second, which is much more likely to cause seizures.

If fits occur it is usually because the person is sensitive to pattern, rather than to flicker, or because a TV screen is being used as a monitor, with the person sitting closer to it than normal.

However, some of my patients have reported having seizures about two or three hours after a long VDU session. There is no real medical explanation for this, but if you notice such an association yourself, it is probably sensible to avoid using a VDU or to use it less frequently or for shorter periods.

CHILDREN AND VIDEO GAMES

Video games are unlikely to induce seizures. The monitors in games arcades have a picture change rate of 70 times a second, and hand-held video games have a liquid crystal display which does not flash in the same way as a VDU. Neither of these is likely to induce photosensitive seizures.

Seizures have sometimes occurred in children who have been playing video games, but in nearly every case it is because a TV screen was used as the monitor, or because the child was sensitive to pattern. Occasionally a specific game is found to trigger seizures; one American manufacturer devised a game which involved 'bad guys' with flashing plates on their chests and backs, and ray guns which were pointed towards the viewer and flashed. Unfortunately, an early trial of the game induced a seizure in a child who was watching it. Further research discovered that the flashes fell well within the sensitivity range of most people with PSE, and the game was withdrawn.

Safety precautions in everyday life

Safety is an important consideration for anyone who has epilepsy. Be sensible, but not so obsessional that your life becomes hedged about with restrictions. Take extra precautions if your seizures are very frequent or severe, and also if you are undergoing a change of drug, when the pattern of your seizures may change.

Around the house

There are some obvious safety measures which you should take if you have generalized tonic clonic seizures: make sure fires are guarded, for example, and take showers rather than baths if you can. If you do take a bath, leave the bathroom door unlocked. Keep bathwater shallow (six inches) and always run in cold water first, then hot, so that if you should have a seizure while sitting on the side of the bath and fall in (it has happened) you will neither scald nor drown yourself.

Sport and exercise

Exercise rarely precipitates a seizure, and unless it happens to do so in your case, there is no reason why you should not take whatever exercise you like, or practise whatever sport you enjoy. It is worth remembering that most people are much less likely to have fits when they are interested and attending to what they are doing. If you have frequent seizures, however, it would obviously be wise not to go in for sports where there would be a high element of risk if you did become unconscious.

Unless they have frequent seizures, or are going through a bad patch, there is no need to stop children taking part in sports such as skateboarding, roller-skating or cycling. It is true that they *might* have a fit and fall off a bicycle, but the chances of this happening are small: road accidents are a hazard to any cyclist.

Let them get their confidence first on minor side roads where traffic is absent or light.

Swimming
Swim only if there are other people with you, and preferably where there is a life-guard – and make sure you tell someone before you go into the water. Wear a brightly-coloured bathing cap so that you are easy to spot if you do run into trouble. Do not swim where the water is murky so that you could not be seen on the bottom, or so deep that you could not be taken out by an ordinary swimmer. Some swimming clubs are very pleased to take people with epilepsy; it is worth shopping around.

Rock climbing and mountaineering
You should only consider these sports if you go into a team with an experienced leader who knows you have epilepsy, and are properly roped.

Parachuting
This is a sport that is best avoided. In any case, without a doctor's certificate you would probably not be allowed to try it, and it is unlikely that any doctor would give you one. However, if you are determined to try it, go for an assisted jump, strapped to an expert who knows you have epilepsy and takes full responsibility for opening the chute and for the landing. Do not go on your own!

Flying
Anyone who has had any sort of fit (apart from febrile convulsions) is disqualified from obtaining a pilot's licence for either commercial or private flying. However, in some special circumstances it may be possible to get your licence back if you have held one in the past and it is at least 10 years since you had a fit. Your examining doctor would have to refer your case to a Civil Aviation Medical Board for their consideration.

There are many people who, despite never having had a seizure, have abnormal epileptic activity in their EEG. At the moment (1995) in Britain pilots are not required to have an EEG and so an abnormal EEG is no bar to gaining a licence.

However many European countries do require commercial pilots to have an EEG and refuse to grant a licence to anyone whose EEG shows abnormal epileptic activity, even if they have never had a seizure. EC regulations may mean that the UK will soon have to comply to European standards; in future commercial pilots probably will require an EEG and if they are discovered to have abnormal EEGs will be refused licences.

Helicopter pilots are always required to have an EEG before being granted a licence. This is because the flicker effect of the helicopter blades is likely to induce seizures in susceptible people (see *photosensitive epilepsy*, pp.124–6).

Gliding

If you have a driving licence the British Gliding Association will probably also allow you to fly gliders, on the grounds that gliding takes place out in the country and even if you do have a fit you are unlikely to damage yourself or anyone else as gliders tend to land safely on their own. My own view would be that you should join a gliding club and go dual until the Chief Flying Instructor is sufficiently happy about your epilepsy and your flying even to discuss a solo flight!

When a parent has epilepsy

'Does mother often do this?' Sue Usiskin's young son was asked by an indignant customer, as Sue lay on the floor after a seizure in a butcher's shop.

Children are going to be exposed to other people's ignorance or intolerance early on and so it is doubly important that the message you give them about epilepsy is a positive one.

Having a parent with epilepsy can have a huge emotional and social impact on a child. How they respond and how well they cope with it will depend more than anything else on how they see their parents behave. Children are great imitators. If their parents' response to a seizure is calm and matter-of-fact, and their attitude is that it is no big deal, then this is the attitude the child is most likely to adopt too.

Parents who have epilepsy need to talk to their children about it, to give them some kind of explanation about what is happening when they have a seizure and to reassure them that it is not dangerous. But many parents do not do this. One survey showed that less than a quarter of parents with epilepsy told their children about it. Sometimes the first a child knows about a parent's epilepsy is when they see that parent having a seizure, a situation which can be very frightening.

Sometimes the problem is that the parents themselves have only a vague understanding of what epilepsy is, and so obviously they find it hard to explain what is wrong to their child. Or they may simply be too embarrassed to talk about it, feeling that their condition is something to be ashamed of and hidden from their children — an attitude which the children themselves will inevitably pick up and reflect.

In some families parents even try to avoid the word epilepsy. They may describe the seizure as a blackout, or a funny turn. Yet these euphemisms may confuse the child even more. Worse still is if the parents decide to tell the child nothing.

The more reluctant parents are to answer questions or give reassurance, the more the child is likely to assume that something is very badly wrong. Inevitably the child will try to piece together an answer for him or herself, and inevitably they will come up with one that is largely based on their own fears. What they imagine to be the truth is almost always infinitely worse than the reality.

Your child's worst fear may be that their parent will die. At the very least, seeing their mother or father taking pills every day, the child is quite likely to assume that they are ill. They may need reassurance that you take medicine not because you are ill, but so that you can stay well. And if your child has seen you having a generalized tonic clonic seizure it is a good thing to tell them quite clearly, even if they do not ask, that seizures are not painful.

If a parent is taken into hospital a young child may worry that they have been abandoned, and that the parent will never return. Children who are told what is happening, and allowed if possible to see or at least speak to the parent while they have to be in hospital, are much less likely to be clingy and insecure when the parent does finally come home.

Older children are often afraid that they too will develop seizures. They need to know that while they may have a higher than average risk, having a parent with seizures does not necessarily mean that they *will* develop seizures themselves.

HELPING CHILDREN COPE

When a parent has epilepsy there may be times when the natural order of things is reversed, and the parent becomes helpless and dependent while the child finds him or herself temporarily in the role of responsible carer in a situation over which he or she has no control. How can you best prepare your child to meet this situation?

One way is to make sure that your child knows what they can do to help if you have a seizure when they are there. Sue Usiskin, who has epilepsy and is an epilepsy counsellor, recommends giving children a simple, practical task to carry out. When her own children were small and she had a seizure, her son would run to get a cloth to place under her face to protect it, while her daughter would sit stroking her face, comforting her. Even very young children can be given some small part to play, and this will make them feel less helpless and less afraid.

Occasionally, in families where the parent finds it difficult to cope with their own seizures, or has severe, disabling epilepsy, the parent may not be able to give the children the emotional support they need. Sometimes this situation leads to a child trying to take on too much responsibility for the parent, so that there is a swopping of roles which may not be healthy for either of them. Children are still children and they need their child-hood; they should not have to take on responsibility for a parent. They need to feel protected and to be looked after themselves. If the parent can not provide this support, it is important that another adult should do so.

Aid in an emergency

One of the special difficulties which anyone who has epilepsy faces is that they may be involved in an accident or found unconscious after a seizure and be given inappropriate treatment by someone who knows nothing of their condition.

Using the Medic-Alert service can help to avoid this danger. Medic-Alert is an organization which runs a special service to protect people with epilepsy. The organization provides a stainless steel bracelet or necklace engraved with the Medic-Alert emblem on one side, and on the reverse, a warning that the wearer has epilepsy, a serial number and an emergency telephone number.

Medic-Alert keep a file with details of your medication, your doctor's phone number, and any other information that may be relevant. In an emergency they will give this information to any doctor or authorized person who telephones them. Calls can be made, reverse charge, at any time and from anywhere in the world. Life membership (which includes the bracelet or necklet) is £13.80.

An alternative is to carry the necessary information about your epilepsy on your person at all times. SOS Talisman make a range of jewellery, which can be bought from most jewellers, incorporating a water-tight locket-style capsule containing an information strip giving your identity and any medical information which would be relevant in an emergency. Or you may prefer just to carry one of the identification cards issued by the British

Epilepsy Association. These are clearly headed *I Have Epilepsy* and give instructions about what should be done if you are discovered unconscious or during a fit.

DEALING WITH AN EPILEPTIC FIT

Most epileptic fits demand no action on the part of the bystander. Even a tonic clonic *grand mal* convulsion is not a medical emergency, though it is frightening to watch, especially if you have never seen one before. All you need to do is to let the fit run its course, making sure that the person is in no physical danger and that their airway is kept clear while they are unconscious. Remember that, however frightening it looks, this may have happened to the person many times before and they have always survived without your help!

What to do

- Don't try to hold the person down or restrain their movements. You may need to move them gently away if they are in immediate danger (by being too near an open fire, for example). Otherwise, simply move any pieces of furniture so that there is a clear space around them, or put padding round any immovable objects which might cause injury.
- **Do not try to force the person's mouth open or wedge anything between their teeth.** They will not choke during the fit and although there is a small risk of them biting their tongue, there is a much greater risk that you will break a tooth by trying to prise their jaws apart. A sore tongue will heal, a broken tooth will not.
- Undo any tight clothing around the person's neck if you can do so easily, and put something soft beneath their head.
- Once the violent movements of the convulsion have stopped, gently turn the person onto their side into the recovery position so that their breathing will not be obstructed while they are unconscious. Wipe any froth from their mouth.

133

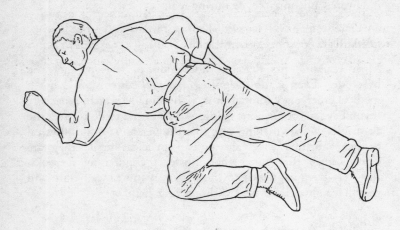

Most people recover quite quickly after a fit, but some need to rest quietly for a while or may even fall deeply asleep. Let the person wake naturally if they are sleeping. Sometimes bladder or bowel control are lost during the fit and one of the most helpful things you can do for someone who has had a seizure is to make sure, when they regain consciousness, that there are clean, dry clothes available for them.

If this is the first time the person has had a fit, they should consult a doctor. But if you are helping someone who has had fits before and is under treatment, there is no need to summon an ambulance or send the person home. Once the seizure is over and they have rested for a while the best thing for them to do is to carry on quite normally and resume whatever they were doing when the fit occurred.

WHEN A SEIZURE IS AN EMERGENCY

Most fits last for only a minute or two. If the convulsions continue for more than five minutes, *or* if another fit begins immediately the first has finished, **summon an ambulance immediately**. Prolonged convulsions, called *status epilepticus*, are dangerous (see p.22). You should call an ambulance, too, if the person does not regain consciousness within a few minutes.

What you should do

- Make sure that the person's airway is clear and they are able to breathe. Put them on their side in the recovery position if you can.
- Gently wipe away any obstructing saliva or froth from their mouth.
- If possible, stay with the person and ask somebody else to call an ambulance immediately. They should say that the person is in *status epilepticus*.
- At the same time as letting the ambulance service know, ring your own doctor in case they can reach you more rapidly than the ambulance.
- If the person has been prescribed rectal valium suppositories (stesolid), give them one of these. If the seizures have not decreased in ten minutes, it would be reasonable to give a second.

Probably the seizures will have stopped by the time the ambulance arrives. However, if they have not, the patient must be given an intravenous injection to stop the seizures. It is therefore important to make sure that the doctor is on his way, as well as the ambulance.

Chapter Nine

Epilepsy, Employment and the Law

Driving regulations in the UK

The risk of accidents is the reason that every country imposes some driving restrictions on people who have epilepsy. If you are diagnosed as having epilepsy, the realization that you will not be able to drive for at least two years may be one of the hardest blows. For many people, losing their driving licence is losing their independence. Recent research suggests that people with epilepsy who drive have the same road traffic accident rate as the average driver, but that they have a higher rate of crashes involving injury. Drivers with epilepsy are also more often involved in fatal road traffic accidents.

No one who suffers from seizures is eligible for a driving licence. In most countries, however, your licence can be renewed once your epilepsy is controlled and you have been seizure-free for a certain length of time. The seizure-free interval required before a driving licence can be issued varies from country to country. In several countries, including Japan, someone with epilepsy is prohibited forever from being granted a driver's licence. In others, the seizure-free time required varies from six to thirty-six months. In the USA each state has its own requirements, varying from six months to two years.

The regulations in the UK have recently been changed to bring us into line with the EC, reducing the fit-free period that is required before a licence can be granted from *two* years to *one*. You are now allowed to hold an ordinary driving licence if you satisfy two of the following three conditions:

	1	You must have been free of fits for at least one year (with or without treatment);
or	2	You have had attacks only whilst asleep for at least three years (with or without treatment);
and	3	Your driving is not likely to be a source of danger to the public.

If you are taking anticonvulsant drugs, it may be that although the treatment means that you satisfy conditions 1 or 2, the drugs themselves impair your driving ability so that you do not satisfy condition 3. Sometimes the side-effects of medication – drowsiness, double vision and slowing in reaction time – mean that even though you are seizure-free there may be risks involved if you are in charge of a vehicle.

Your fitness to drive will be assessed by your doctor, and he or she will take into account the effects of the drugs that control your seizures as well as the degree of seizure control that you have achieved. In the UK (though not in some other countries, for example some states in the USA) your doctor has no legal responsibility to inform the Licensing Authority that you have epilepsy. It is up to you to do this, though your doctor must make sure that you know you have to do so. Your doctor will only break confidentiality and inform the Licensing Authority if he or she believes that is in your or the public's best interests, and if you consistently refuse to inform the Licensing Authority yourself.

The type of epilepsy you have or the severity of your seizures makes no difference; *any* seizure symptoms (apart from seizures during sleep) can prevent you gaining a licence. However, it is the Director of the Driving Licence Authority at Swansea who has the last word. If he rules against you, you can, if you wish, appeal, and your case would be heard in front of a magistrate. It is highly unlikely that a magistrate would overrule Swansea unless there were exceptional circumstances.

If a licence is granted, it will be made dependent on your continuing treatment. If your treatment is altered, or stopped, then you will have to stop driving until your doctor and the Driving Licence Authority are again satisfied that it is safe for you to drive. You will also be required to apply for a new licence every three years. However, under a recent new policy, drivers with epilepsy who have been seizure-free for six years and who are not at risk of progressive epilepsy can now be granted licences until the age of 70.

The regulations for drivers of buses and heavy goods vehicles are more strict. Driving is not permitted if a person is 'liable to epileptic seizures'. This wording is generally interpreted as meaning that the person should have been free from seizures for at least ten years; that during this seizure-free period they should not have taken anti-epileptic medication; and that there should no longer be any likelihood of them having seizures. This would exclude anyone who has any brain damage which has previously caused seizures.

Train drivers
The restrictions are even more severe for train drivers. No one who has had even one fit after the age of five can become a train driver. In the case of London Underground, anyone who has ever had a fit is excluded.

Insurance
Most types of insurance are available for people with epilepsy, but the premiums may be higher.

Epilepsy and employment

There were two schools of thought about employers and epilepsy, Tom would say when any of his friends asked him if he had had any luck getting a job yet. One is that if you don't tell them you have epilepsy and they find out you'll get sacked on the spot. The other is that if you do tell them, the chances are that they won't employ you anyway. Tom was quite clear about where he stood. He was an up-front sort of chap, and he didn't like anything that smacked of deception. So he always made it quite clear to any prospective employer that he had had epilepsy since he was a small boy and that he had to take drugs all the time to control it – in fact that he was likely to be quite a liability to any firm willing to employ him.

The next time Tom went to see his doctor, he was asked the same question: 'Isn't it time you got a job, Tom? It's over two years since you left school. You can't spend the rest of your life hanging about.' Tom was aggrieved. You couldn't say he hadn't tried. But he had to be honest about his epilepsy, didn't he? Otherwise it wouldn't be fair.

'That's all very well, Tom,' said his doctor. 'But don't you think you might paint a slightly rosier picture for a prospective employer? Can I remind you that your seizures are well under control? You haven't had one in two years, have you? And two seizure-free years means that you don't actually have epilepsy. You could do pretty much any job you wanted to – I'm assuming you don't want to be a steeplejack. Is it possible that you are actually not too keen to find a job? Think about it . . .'

If your seizures are well controlled, there is no reason why you should not work, or why you should have to seek 'safe' or sheltered employment, why you should be passed over for promotion, or why you should not work near machinery.

Prejudice and misconceptions about epilepsy account for most of the difficulties you may have in getting employment. For example, although the drugs you are taking may make you less alert, your epilepsy itself will not affect your ability to handle machines. Much is made of the dangers of falling forward onto machinery during a fit, but in fact most people who fall during a fit fall *backwards*, not forwards.

Unless your epilepsy is very severe or caused by serious brain damage there is no reason why your employment prospects should be limited. Probably about 85 per cent of people who have epilepsy should be able to find employment in normal jobs in the normal way. One study from Canada showed that when local doctors, social workers and epilepsy associations were prepared to support local business firms, it was very much easier for people with epilepsy to obtain employment, partly because such co-operation led to greater understanding and lack of prejudice. More important, local employers found that employees with epilepsy were more likely to be reliable as they valued their jobs and did not want to lose them.

RESTRICTIONS IN EMPLOYMENT

There are only a few occupations you will not be able to follow, including heavy goods vehicle or public service driving (see above), becoming a commercial pilot or joining the armed services. A few potentially hazardous jobs, such as a steeplejack or deep-sea diver are also obviously precluded.

You will not be able to become a merchant seaman if you have had any history of fits after the age of 5 years. If you are already a merchant seaman and then develop epilepsy you will be able to continue your employment once you have remained seizure-free for at least two years provided that you are working on a ship carrying a medical officer and are not directly involved with the safety of the ship or passengers.

If you are currently having seizures you cannot be recruited for the police, or as a traffic warden. However, those with a past history of epilepsy are considered individually. Applicants for teacher training should have been free from seizures for two years at the time of applying.

SEEKING HELP

If your epilepsy is disabling, and you have problems finding work, you can seek help from the PACT – Placing, Assessment and Counselling Team. PACT can be contacted through your local Job Centre. One of their specially trained Disability Employment Advisors will help you decide what job you want to do and help you find it, and offer advice on a wide range of services, including job training, rehabilitation courses, and travel grants for getting to and from work.

VOLUNTARY WORK

If you have been trying, and failing, to get work for some time, it is worth thinking about the possibility of doing unpaid voluntary work for a while. This keeps you in touch with people and with the working world, and may also give you experience which will be valuable in your future job-seeking. Your local Council for Voluntary Services or Social Services office are the people to contact if the idea of voluntary work appeals to you.

APPLYING FOR A JOB

When you are applying for a new job, you have to keep two clear aims in mind. First you must convince your prospective employer that you are perfectly capable of doing the job in question. Second, you must make them believe that your epilepsy does not play a particularly important part in your life; that for you it is no big deal.

Unfortunately, many people with epilepsy have learnt through bitter experience that even to mention that you have epilepsy may lose them the job, but that *not* mentioning it may eventually have the same effect. It can be a no-win situation, but perhaps the best approach is to sell yourself and your abilities before even mentioning the fact that you have epilepsy. So do not mention it on your application form, unless you are specifically asked, or even during the initial phase of the interview. It should be your final disclosure, and when you make it, do so briefly and casually, as an aside. Then, if your interviewer asks you any further questions, answer them as honestly and straightforwardly as you can.

'I take the attitude,' one woman says, 'that if a firm don't want to employ me and my epilepsy, then I'm sure I don't want to work for them.'

PENSION SCHEMES

The fact that you have epilepsy should make no difference to your inclusion in your employer's pension scheme. The general advice of the Occupational Pensions Board is that if someone is suitable for a job, then they are also suitable for inclusion in the pension scheme.

ACCIDENT INSURANCE

Employers' liability policies cover all employees. Those with epilepsy are no exception. Provided you have declared your epilepsy and you are not employed in a job for which your epilepsy makes you quite unsuitable, accident insurance should not be a problem for you or your employer.

10

Children With Epilepsy

'*T*erry was seven when she had her first grand mal *seizure. The best way I can describe what it was like is to say, how would you feel if you could see your child* **dying** *in front of your eyes? I know now that she wasn't in any danger, but that's not what it seemed like at the time. Then, when the doctor told us she had epilepsy, I thought, how could this happen to us? We've never been a family to worry much about our health, but then you don't appreciate it till you have to face the fact that someone's ill. I thought, she's going to have this for the rest of her life. She's never going to be able to live a normal life, like other children. And me, I'm going to have to look after her. What's it going to do to me?*'

How do you feel when you discover that your child has epilepsy? Most parents are overwhelmed by all kinds of feelings: grief for their child, fears for his or her safety and doubts about their own ability to cope. It may feel as though the high hopes that you, like every parent, have for your child have been dashed. Anger is a common reaction: why did this have to happen to our family, to our child? You may even feel resentful at the disruptive effect the discovery has made on your own life and your own plans. And however irrational it is, you are very likely to feel guilty, as though the whole thing is somehow your fault, something that you should have been able to prevent.

These initial feelings are normal and natural, and you are likely to have them however much you love your child. Eventually they will lessen, especially if you have a doctor who is willing to answer your questions and give you the information and reassurance you need, and if as a couple you and your partner can help each other through this stage, sharing the worry and the responsibility.

It often helps to talk to other parents who have experienced what you are going through. Joining a support group can be very comforting and also a helpful and important source of information. The British Epilepsy Association (see Appendix) will be able to tell you if there is an epilepsy support group in your area.

Diagnosing children with epilepsy

There are special difficulties in diagnosing the child with epilepsy. Children, and especially adolescents, do behave strangely at times. At school, children with absence seizures may be accused of day-dreaming or lack of concentration, considered disobedient or inattentive. In adolescents especially, the irrational and sometimes truculent behaviour associated with partial complex seizures is often mistaken for a disorder of behaviour.

But equally, there are serious consequences for the child if he or she is mistakenly diagnosed as having epilepsy when what they are actually suffering from is some other episode of disturbed behaviour. Breath-holding attacks and night terrors in young children, temper tantrums, fainting in school assembly and migraine are all sometimes confused with epilepsy.

One of the most difficult things about epilepsy is its unpredictability and uncertainty. Even when your child has been diagnosed as having epilepsy, it may take some weeks before the pattern of their fits has been worked out, and the best medication for them has been found. You will want to know what the long-term prospects are for your child, and whether he or she will outgrow their epilepsy, and these are predictions that your doctor may be reluctant to make straight away. If there is a strong family history of epilepsy, the chances are good that your child will improve after adolescence or even that they will outgrow their epilepsy by the time they are 16.

Helping the child with epilepsy

All parents are anxious about their children. It is perhaps inevitable that if you have a child with epilepsy you will be especially anxious and concerned. There is a risk that, probably without realizing it, you may become so over-concerned about them and so protective that you hamper their social development, restrict their personality, and isolate them from other children. Epilepsy in itself is not a bar to happiness. But the child with no friends will certainly not be happy.

No child likes to feel different. Perhaps the greatest danger of childhood epilepsy is that it will permanently lower the child's self-esteem, by making them feel they are in some way handicapped or less of a complete person.

How your child feels about having epilepsy will depend very much on how you react. All children need to feel valued and feel good about themselves, because the way they see themselves colours their actions and behaviour. Children who have a positive view of themselves tend to do better in school, to have more friends, and to have a sense of competence about their own lives – a belief that they are at least to some extent in control of what happens to them.

It is quite easy for children who have epilepsy to grow up without this positive view of themselves. Children tend to adopt their parents' view of them, and children who have epilepsy will see themselves through their parents' eyes, and adopt their parents' views about the epilepsy.

TALKING ABOUT EPILEPSY

In many families, epilepsy is something that is just not talked about. One study has shown that in only half of the families where a child had epilepsy were brothers and sisters told of the diagnosis. Even the child themselves may not be told. Obviously a child has to be told something, simply because they have to be given some reason to co-operate in the treatment they have to undergo. But often they are given information only in the vaguest of terms. Sometimes parents will say that they think the child knows he or she has epilepsy, even though it is not talked about. Sometimes even when the child asks the parents directly, he or she gets an evasive answer, because the parents feel they cannot speak openly and frankly about it.

If parents are clearly unwilling to talk about the epilepsy, the danger is that they will convey the impression that it is 'bad', and their child will come to see it as something to be ashamed of, which has to be concealed. Unfortunately many parents clearly *do* contrive to convey this attitude. A conspiracy of silence is a bad start for anyone who has to live with the condition.

Children's fears about epilepsy
This conspiracy of silence means that the children involved can not talk to anyone about their epilepsy. If they have questions, these will not be answered, and also if they do have anxieties, they can not be reassured.

What most usually concerns them is the cause of their seizures, and the effects seizures may have. They worry about having seizures in the future, and about the way that epilepsy may restrict their activities and their lives.

Sometimes children are frightened to go to sleep in case they have a seizure. They may ask, 'Why me? What did I do to deserve seizures?' Some feel guilty because they know their parents are worried. Some have fears of being mentally ill.

A major worry is about being teased at school, or by their brothers or sisters. Some children say they feel different from their peers and worry about a seizure occurring when with friends. If this does happen they are especially likely to be fearful about going to school.

How to tell a child they have epilepsy
First find out as much as you can from your doctor about the kind of epilepsy that your child has, and its likely outcome.

When you tell the child they have epilepsy, do not make it seem a major disaster, or even a drama. Be straightforward and matter of fact. Give it a name: epilepsy. Do not resort to calling it 'funny turns' or worse still, not naming it at all. This is very confusing for a child. Stress that epilepsy is not really an illness because between seizures the child is perfectly well. And point out that they have to take medicine every day, not because they are ill, but to help them stay well.

Be guided by your child and let them ask the questions. Children may not be able to take in too much information to begin with. At first, simple reassurance may be all that is needed. If the child is young it will probably be enough just to tell them they have epilepsy, reassure them that it is no big deal, and explain that they need to take medicine to stop the attacks.

An older child will probably want more information, so you should try to be as well informed as possible so that you can answer their questions. Encourage them to ask questions, and if you do not know the answers, be honest and make a note to ask your doctor at the next appointment.

If you feel anxious about talking to your child, it might help you to contact the British Epilepsy Association, or your local Epilepsy Support Group, and ask if there is a counsellor in your area who could be with you when you tell your child and help answer any questions. If this is someone who has epilepsy themselves, so much the better.

Telling other people
Grandparents and other relatives, friends and neighbours, the child's own teachers and friends, indeed anyone who comes into close contact with your child or looks after them may also need to be told. When you explain to other people about your child's epilepsy, what kind of reaction can you expect? Usually you will receive sympathy and support. When you do meet a more doubtful reaction it is more often due to ignorance and fear than outright prejudice. Talking to someone who knows rather more than they do may be enough to dispel it. Some parents have found that older people (even grandparents) are more ignorant, and therefore more likely to react in this way than people of their own generation.

DO NOT LET EPILEPSY TAKE OVER

The best thing you can do for your child is to treat them as normally as possible and make sure they lead as normal a life as they can. Encourage them to play with other children and never feel you must keep them continually under your eye in case they have a fit. After all, in terms of time, the child's fits occupy only a tiny part of their life. So try, if you can, to keep your own concern in proportion.

Letting epilepsy take too high a profile in the family's life is almost as bad as ignoring the fact that a child has seizures. Your child's epilepsy is only one of the many aspects of their individuality. It is certainly not the one they would want to become identified with. If 'epileptic' is always the label they feel they are given, they may come to think of their epilepsy as the most significant thing about them, and other people may come to perceive them in this way too. That kind of labelling can take years to live down.

Do not assume that if your child is difficult or behaves badly, this is all due to the epilepsy. *All* children are sometimes aggressive, inattentive, badly behaved, restless or rude. Those few children whose epilepsy is due to brain damage, particularly to lesions in the temporal lobe (especially the left temporal lobe), do seem to be more prone to behaviour disorders. But on the whole, your child's behaviour will depend on their relationship to you, and your attitude towards their epilepsy. There is no good evidence to suggest that bad behaviour is a characteristic of children with uncomplicated epilepsy. Epilepsy should never be made an excuse for bad behaviour.

Try not to give the child too much special treatment or make them the centre of attention. Many parents worry about giving a child with epilepsy the ordinary discipline or sanctions that they would give other children in the family without a second thought, in case they provoke a seizure. But you must avoid training your child to use seizures as a defence or a distraction whenever things get difficult or they are under stress.

You are doing your child no favours by letting them use their epilepsy as an excuse if things go wrong. Life can be frustrating and difficult and the child with epilepsy has to get used to the ordinary frustrations of life just like any other child.

RISK TAKING

All child-rearing involves allowing your child to take some risks. All children have to explore and to experiment, to test their limits, to find out what they can or can not do. Children with epilepsy are no exception. If they are to grow and develop successfully they need freedom to make at least a certain number of their own mistakes. Of course you have to minimize the physical risks, but it is much better to teach your children to assess risks for themselves. Encourage your child to take sensible precautions and work out his or her own ways of staying safe rather than trying to wrap them in cotton wool so that they never have to face hazards and use their own judgment. You have to learn to strike a balance between protecting them and encouraging them to do any activity that might help their own development.

There is no reason why children with epilepsy should not play team games, for example. Swimming is an acceptable risk too, *provided a child's seizures are well controlled and a competent life-saver is on hand* (see p.128). Whether cycling is sensible depends largely on the type of epilepsy the child has; you may feel in any case that it is wisest to allow cycling only off main roads. Though it must depend on the type of epilepsy and the frequency of seizures, there need be no reason why a child with epilepsy should not use a climbing frame, or climb a tree that is not too tall.

Taking medication

It is essential that your child learns to take their drugs regularly, every day at the right time. Most children are surprisingly co-operative about this. A good aid to memory for anyone, child or adult, who has to take long-term medication is a 'dosette' which you can buy from your chemist. This is a container which has seven removable compartments, labelled with the days of the week. Each compartment has four slots, so that it can take four doses of medication. The dosette is filled with the appropriate daily doses of anticonvulsant at the beginning of each week and at any time you can see at a glance whether the child has or has not remembered to take their tablets. If they have to go away for a day or two they simply take the dosette container for those days with them.

All anticonvulsants have some side-effects (see p.43). But although the drugs your child is given may affect their ability to concentrate, proper treatment with the appropriate drugs should not have a serious effect on your child's learning or behaviour. If you think your child is being badly affected by their drugs, you must tell your doctor. Although much better drugs with fewer side-effects are now available, phenobarbitone and the related drug primidone (which often cause restlessness, irritability or mental slowing) are still sometimes prescribed for children. If your child has been prescribed one of these anticonvulsants, discuss the possibility of a change with your doctor. If he feels a change is not necessary or advisable seek a second opinion. These drugs should be avoided wherever possible for children of school age.

Whenever a new drug is prescribed for your child, watch carefully for any change in their behaviour and report it to your doctor; the new drug may not suit them.

The child with epilepsy at school

Most children with epilepsy go to a normal school and do well. When your child starts at any new school you should talk to their new teachers, who may have very old-fashioned or mistaken ideas about what someone with epilepsy can or can not safely be allowed to do.

Explain to the school about your child's epilepsy, and tell his or her teachers what will happen if they have a seizure. Tell the matron what drugs the child is on. Usually schools are understanding and co-operative, and a headteacher will pass on to the teachers in charge of the child whatever information you give them. But just occasionally they fail to do so. If the school is large and you get the feeling that the headteacher is insufficiently concerned, it would probably be worthwhile talking to your child's class teacher yourself, just to make sure that the information filters down to the right level.

The child's own friends usually accept the fact that he or she has seizures quite matter of factly. A few children do get teased, but teasing is often not as big a problem as most parents expect it to be. Some children even find that their seizures make them more interesting to their peers.

Your child's teachers probably see almost as much of them as you do and an observant and co-operative teacher is a valuable asset. They may recognize changes in your child's behaviour or physical state even before you do. Always ask them to discuss any changes they do notice with you; these changes may be an indication that your child's medication needs adjusting.

WHAT TO TELL THE TEACHERS

- Make it clear to the school that you want your child to take part in the whole range of the school's activities. There is no reason why they should not play games, for example, or swim (see *Sport and exercise*, pp.127–9); in fact (except in rare cases) there is every reason why they *should* do these things.
- Explain to teachers that there is usually no need to send your child home after an attack unless they have been hurt. It is enough just to allow them to sit quietly for a while to recover, before carrying on with normal school activities.
- Get a clear and realistic assessment from your doctor about what your child should be capable of. It is a good idea, too, to ask your doctor to arrange for the child to be tested by a psychologist so that you know what his level of intelligence is and where his skills or difficulties lie. Once a child is labelled an 'epileptic' there is a real danger that their teachers may underestimate their academic potential and give them neither stimulation nor encouragement. The child who is expected to do badly almost certainly will do badly.
- Keep a positive attitude. Emphasize what the child *can* do, not what they can not. Help them to develop social skills so that they are a likeable person.
- Make sure that the staff are prepared to treat your child as far as possible just like the other children, both in

terms of punishment as well as reward. Teachers may be tempted to let them get away with too much because they are afraid that discipline or reprimand might cause a seizure. Such special treatment will not make your child popular with the other children.

- Keep the child's attendance at school as regular as you can. The reason many children with epilepsy do badly is simply because they have missed so much schooling.

TAKING MEDICATION AT SCHOOL

Most children with epilepsy are able to take their medication twice daily, outside school hours. But a few may need a dose during the school day. And very occasionally, staff may have to give emergency treatment with rectal diazepam to a child in *status epilepticus.*

If your child needs to take a dose of anticonvulsant during school hours, make sure that the school has written details about how and when the medicine is to be taken, whether it should be given by a named teacher (in which case the parent should give written permission) or whether the child is to be responsible for their own medication. Secondary school children (unless they have learning difficulties that would make it impossible) should be responsible for taking their own medication. Younger children should be encouraged to be self-reliant too, but it will depend very much on how responsible the child is generally, and whether the school is prepared to allow them this particular responsibility. If the medicine is to be stored (for example, if the school is to keep rectal diazepam for emergency use) you need to agree with the school who is responsible for giving it (they may need special training) and where it is to be kept for easy access if it is needed. Label all medication with the child's name and the dose and frequency of its administration.

In the current climate, many teachers are uneasy about giving rectal diazepam to a child. To protect teachers against the possibility that they might be vulnerable to allegations of child abuse in these circumstances, two adults should be present if rectal diazepam has to be given to a child.

CHILDREN WHO DO NOT ACHIEVE

When your child is first diagnosed as having epilepsy, one of your first concerns is likely to be about the effect the epilepsy will have on their intelligence and mental ability.

Some children who have epilepsy do, undoubtedly, fail to achieve what they should be capable of at school. But once again, this is nearly always a by-product of the epilepsy and not a direct result of it. Sometimes children underachieve because they have fallen behind in their school work through frequent absences, more often underachievement is due to the drugs they are on (see above), though probably a major factor is also the attitude of parents and the school towards children with epilepsy. For everyone's sake, ask for your child to be properly assessed by a neuropsychologist (see p.29) so that you and the school have a realistic idea of what they should be capable of, and in which subjects they are likely to have difficulties. If the school is unable to organize this itself, ask your doctor to arrange it by referring your child to the local mental health services for psychometric (IQ and skill measurement) assessment.

Whether epilepsy does cause mental deterioration has been a matter of debate for over 100 years. Rapid diagnosis and assessment of the epilepsy after the onset of the first seizure, and good control of seizures seem to be the most important factors involved. If there is mental decline, it is likely to be most noticeable in the first years (or perhaps even the first few months) after the onset of epilepsy. This initial phase is followed by a stable phase with little further deterioration.

Practical safety tips

- Get an engaged notice to hang on the outside of bathroom and lavatory doors instead of locking them.
- Baths are a potential hazard for anyone who has seizures. Showers are safer. When baths are taken, always run in cold water first, then add hot, so that the water never reaches a dangerously hot temperature. Bathwater should be kept shallow: about six inches is safest.
- A regular routine with regular meals and plenty of sleep is important for any child, but especially so for the child who has epilepsy.
- Do not leave your child alone after a seizure. They may be confused and need comfort and reassurance. If the seizure seems worse or different from usual, contact your doctor immediately.
- Make sure the child always carries something (a Medic-Alert bracelet, for example) with their name and address and the information that they have epilepsy.

FEBRILE CONVULSIONS

Children's brains are more excitable, and therefore more seizure-prone than adults. Between three and six per cent of children sometimes have convulsions when running a high temperature. These febrile convulsions tend to run in families. They usually last only a few seconds or, at the most, a minute or two, and take the form of a *grand mal* seizure. Febrile convulsions are nearly always harmless for the child, though frightening to watch. Most children grow out of them by the time they are two or three years old.

However, children run a greater risk than adults of developing *status epilepticus* (prolonged or repeated convulsions) during a fit. This *is* dangerous, and may cause permanent brain damage and even, occasionally, be fatal. About five per cent of children who have febrile convulsions go on to develop epilepsy later in life. This is probably because during severe febrile convulsions the brain has been damaged through a partial deprivation of oxygen. The damaged area is usually the temporal lobe, which is the part of the brain most vulnerable to lack of oxygen. There is some recent evidence to suggest that a few children are born with an abnormality in this part of the brain which causes them to have severe febrile convulsions. But whatever the cause, the result is that after a severe febrile convulsion these children are left with an area of damage in the temporal lobe which later acts as a focus for seizures.

It is therefore important that febrile convulsions should be treated quickly; always call your doctor or an ambulance if your child develops a convulsion during a fever. Once your child has had one febrile convulsion, your GP will want to take steps to ensure they do not have another. Some years ago most doctors believed that children who have a tendency to febrile convulsions should be given regular anticonvulsant medication, usually Epilim (sodium valproate), to prevent fits until they have outgrown the tendency. The view now is more flexible, and practice varies quite widely. It is most likely that your doctor will not give regular medication after a first febrile convulsion unless it was very prolonged and led to the child being kept in hospital for a day or two. Some doctors will not even give medication after a second or third febrile convulsion, but wait for a trend to be established before giving regular anticonvulsants.

When your doctor makes the decision, one of the most important guiding factors will be whether there is a strong family history of febrile convulsions which have not led to the development of epilepsy. A strong family history is usually seen as a sign of a child being likely to outgrow the convulsions without permanent damage, and so the need for medication is less.

In addition, your doctor will probably suggest that if your child has had a fit in the past, you should give them paracetamol whenever they start to run a temperature, and sponge them with tepid water to help bring the temperature down. The fact that your child has a tendency to have febrile convulsions and may even have to take an anticonvulsant drug does not mean that they have epilepsy; the treatment is just to prevent further convulsions which might eventually cause epilepsy.

A few children may have a short-lived paralysis down one side of the body after a severe febrile convulsion. If this happens, it is worthwhile noting and remembering which side of the body is affected. Some of these children may later go on to develop temporal lobe epilepsy; if they do, and if it is thought they might benefit from surgery, it can be very helpful to the doctor to know which side was paralysed at the time of that early seizure. The side of the paralysis is a very good indication of the side of the brain in which the seizure focus is likely to lie.

Parents' concerns

In a recent survey, parents of children who had epilepsy were asked to list the things that concerned them most. Their top ten worries were these:

1 Whether their child might die in a seizure

The chances of this happening are very small. I can not say that they are non-existent because, very rarely, people unfortunately do die during a prolonged *grand mal* seizure. However they are usually young male adults, very seldom children. With any other type of seizure the risk is negligible.

Worrying that death during a seizure *might* happen will make your life miserable. Instead make sure that you know what to do if your child does have a prolonged convulsion (see p.135), so that if an emergency arises it does not turn into a catastrophe.

2 Whether the child will suffer brain damage or become insane

Seizures themselves, provided they are not prolonged, do not cause brain damage, though it is possible for a child who has such severe seizures that they frequently fall over to suffer head injury and subsequent brain damage.

3 Whether the child might become insane

Seizures do not lead to mental illness, with the exception of a few adults and even fewer children who develop a very rare complication of a short mental illness after a run of generalized seizures. This illness usually only lasts for one or two weeks before the child returns to normal. However, it is such a very rare occurrence that it should not even figure on your worry-scale.

4 Guilt, because parents think that they may have done something to cause the condition

It is very common for parents whose children have epilepsy to blame themselves. You have to remind yourself that you had no responsibility for your own genetic make-up and thus no responsibility for the genes that you pass on to your children. It is no one's fault; it is just the way things are. Overcoming these feelings of guilt is all part of you coming to terms with your child's epilepsy. Unless you do come to terms with it you cannot help your child to do so.

5 Frustration at not knowing the cause of the seizures, especially if they have been given no adequate explanation

This is a situation which really need not arise nowadays. It is certainly much less common than it used to be, because of the marked improvement in neuroimaging technology which allows a much more detailed view of the structure of the brain and its function. Doctors can now discover the cause of epilepsy in about 90 per cent of cases. Even if you have not been told the cause of your child's epilepsy, the chances are that your doctor knows. If he does not, ask to be referred to a specialist.

6 Worry about the development of emotional or behavioural problems in the child

Some children with epilepsy do behave badly and have emotional problems. So do some children without epilepsy. Remember that this kind of problem is not usually due to the epilepsy alone. It is more likely to be caused by the way the child's epilepsy is handled in the family and at school, by the attitude of other children, or by the medication that the child is taking. These are all factors over which you have some control. Never assume that any problem your child has is because of their epilepsy. If you do, you may never look for the true cause, which may be bullying by classmates, an unsympathetic teacher or falling behind in schoolwork – any one of the myriad of reasons that any child has for periods of unhappiness, and which can lead them to behave badly. Once you have found the reason, enlist the help of your doctor or the school in tackling the problem.

7 The impact that the epilepsy may have on the child's future career

There are only a few clear-cut limitations on the employment of anyone who has epilepsy. Your child may never become an HGV driver or a pilot, for example (see pp.139–42), but, on the whole, predictions about a child's future career can only be made when the cause of their epilepsy is known and they have had a proper assessment by a neuropsychologist. Once you know what their intellectual attainment should be, and what their strengths and weaknesses are, you will be in a better position to help your child make realistic choices about their future.

8 The stigma of epilepsy, and the prejudice the child may have to face

Unfortunately no one can control other people's ill-founded beliefs and prejudices. Your child is bound to meet them sometime; what matters is your child's ability to believe that prejudice is the result of ignorance or stupidity and is no reflection on them personally. Your child will largely adopt and reflect your own attitudes. If you have always tried to talk frankly about their epilepsy and give them a positive attitude towards it, you will go a long way to counterbalance other people's prejudices.

9 School problems, especially the effects on learning and memory of epilepsy and medication

Epilepsy and, more usually, the drugs used to treat it, can have an effect on learning and memory (see *Drugs*, pp.42–58). Sometimes a change of medication can make a huge difference, so talk to your doctor if you think the drugs your child is taking are slowing them down. When your child goes to junior school, and again when they enter secondary school at 11, they should be assessed by a neuropsychologist so that everyone concerned knows what the child is capable of and, without having unrealistic expectations of them, encourages them to reach their full potential. Some children will do very well and have no difficulty; others may need special help. (see *Children who do not achieve*, above).

10 The difficulty parents find in having a social life outside the family

This problem may operate on several different levels. It may be that the child can not be left by the parents. Or it may be that the parents feel that they can not leave their child – a very different matter. The obstacle may also be the parents' feelings about the way other people view them; they may feel so uncomfortable or defensive about their child's epilepsy that it makes social contact difficult for them. Or it may simply be that the parents' lives have become so bound up with caring for their child that they have little time to keep up old friendships or to make new ones. They may, in fact, have got out of the habit of having a social life.

There are partial solutions to all these problems, though it is unrealistic not to accept that without help or the means to buy help in, it can be very difficult for those few parents whose children have very severe epilepsy to develop some sort of life of their own. Social services may be able to arrange respite care, and some social services benefits may allow you to employ help and thus get some freedom.

That said, the vast majority of families never face anything like such a difficult situation. Often there is no reason why a child with epilepsy can not spend time apart from their parents if sensible arrangements are made with a friend, relative or baby-sitter. Parents may feel guilty about being away from their child, or may feel no one else is capable of looking after their child properly, but these feelings are usually unrealistic. Epilepsy support groups are a good way for parents to wean themselves out of the house into an environment where other people will be understanding and sympathetic to the way they feel. A child's epilepsy can not and should not become the whole focus of the parent's life. It is not fair on the parents, neither is it good for the child.

The adolescent with epilepsy

'Mum used to get really mad at me. I did everything I wasn't supposed to – partied all night, missed meals, drank too much. And I wasn't too good at taking my pills either, though I have to admit there were other drugs I took pretty regularly! I knew exactly what I was doing, and I knew it wasn't doing my epilepsy much good either. It certainly made me have more seizures. But somehow that didn't matter too much – what was more important to me was to feel I wasn't missing out on anything, that I was doing what my mates were doing. I didn't want to have epilepsy. I didn't want to be different. I suppose I've got a bit more sense now, but I don't regret it. I had a good time then.'

This is how Adrian, now 22 and leading a rather more sober and regular life, his seizures well under control, described his teenage years. Adrian was lucky; his epilepsy was not too bad and his seizures never went seriously out of control. His behaviour might have had dangerous consequences if his epilepsy had been more severe.

Adolescence is a difficult time for any teenager. For the teenager with epilepsy (especially if the condition develops during adolescence) it can be particularly difficult. Their own good health is something that most teenagers are able to take so much for granted that it is not even a matter for thought, let alone a cause for concern. The teenager with epilepsy may become suddenly and uncomfortably aware of the fact that they are 'different' – the last thing any adolescent wants to be. Their self-esteem may take a dive and they are beset not only by anxiety about the seizures themselves, but about what they look like during a seizure and the loss of dignity involved in having a seizure in front of their friends. They have to cope with social difficulties too: when they meet a new girlfriend or boyfriend, should they tell them about the epilepsy? And if so should they broach the subject early on in the friendship, or wait till they know each other better?

WHOSE EPILEPSY IS IT ANYWAY?

How much independence a teenager should be given, and how soon, causes more friction between parents and adolescents than almost anything else. When a child has epilepsy it can be especially difficult for the parents to stand back and let the child make their own decisions and, sometimes, their own mistakes. But this letting go has to happen if the child is eventually to become independent.

One of the ways you can encourage your child to become independent is by helping them build up their own relationship with their doctor and encouraging them to ask their own questions. As your child enters their teens, make sure you do not go with them every time they have an appointment with their doctor. Letting them go on their own is a first step towards letting them take over responsibility for their epilepsy along with other areas of their life.

HOW TEENAGERS COPE

Not surprisingly, many teenagers find it very hard to come to terms with a diagnosis of epilepsy. What is more surprising is that it seems to be those adolescents who have tonic clonic seizures but have never had a seizure in public, and those who have simple epilepsy with no complications and no significant brain damage, who seem to find it most difficult to cope. Their most potent anxiety seems to be the fear of 'coming out' – of being recognized as having epilepsy. Teenagers who are to all intents and purposes perfectly normal and healthy and whose friends may have no idea they have epilepsy may feel they have everything to lose if their condition is 'discovered'. So it is perhaps not so surprising that the diagnosis hits them so hard.

Coping by acting out

Anxiety and stress often show themselves in generally difficult, 'acting-out' behaviour. There may be verbal abuse, temper tantrums or aggressive outbursts. Or there may be more serious problems: suicide gestures, drug abuse or running away from home. Your child may refuse to talk or listen to you, but they do need to talk to someone, and it may be easier for them if that someone is not directly involved, especially if they can talk to them in confidence. Professional help is called for.

If you are a parent faced with this problem, the best place to start is with your GP. Some GP practices have their own counselling service. If yours does not, contact the British Epilepsy Association and ask if there is an epilepsy counsellor in your area. Finally, you could ask your GP to refer your child to the local psychiatric services specifically for counselling.

Coping by regression

Adolescence is the time when children should start to become independent, taking control of their own life and making their own friends and their own decisions. This is an essential part of growing up. Young teenagers who develop epilepsy often react by regressing, becoming more childlike and dependent. This

kind of behaviour is almost bound to increase their parents'
natural tendency to be overprotective towards them. The child
may then find him or herself in an uncomfortable situation – on
the one hand hostile because they hate being controlled and
resent it; on the other hand feeling dependent on the very people
who are arousing this hostility. There is a real danger that the
normal development of the adolescent into an adult will be
hindered, and that for too long they will remain unnaturally
dependent on their parents.

Coping by denial

One quite common reaction is for the teenager to deny that
anything is wrong. Often such denial is self-destructive: they
may stop taking their medication or refuse to go for their regular
clinic check-ups. But it can also be the way they protect
themselves from the ridicule of other people. For someone
whose epilepsy is well controlled, ignoring the epilepsy's existence may seem easier than 'coming out' and explaining it to
friends.

Unfortunately there are features of the adolescent's life style
(late nights and shortage of sleep, irregular meals, emotional
stress and alcohol abuse) which are likely to be especially harmful
to someone with epilepsy. A teenager who is determined to lead
an ordinary teenage life despite their epilepsy may develop what
parents see as a wilful disregard of their own health and safety.
Throughout their teenage years, adolescents become increasingly
reluctant to let parents interfere in or control their life. For
parents of a child with epilepsy, who know that their child's
health is on the line, giving up control is particularly hard.

It is difficult for parents to get the balance right. Limits still
have to be set, and it is impossible for them to stand by and do
nothing. And yet too many remonstrations about risk-taking
behaviour, too many reminders about taking medication and
keeping appointments may be counter-productive.

It is worth reminding yourself that all teenagers are at least a
little rebellious, and all are struggling to get a measure of
independence from their parents. The only strategy which is

likely to work is to give your son or daughter as much control and independence as you can in other ways. Do not waste your energy or influence on things which really do not matter so much or which are none of your business: their friendships, for example, the clothes they wear or the hairstyles they adopt. There is then rather more chance that they will be prepared to listen to you about the things which really are important, and that they may perhaps even modify their behaviour.

Children whose attitude is to deny their epilepsy also refuse to regard it as a handicap. They do not allow it to prevent them doing what they want, or to impede their development and their plans for the future. This is a healthy attitude to take, but they should also be realistic in their ambitions. Occasionally denial can lead to self-destructive behaviour – for example when a teenager decides that they are perfectly capable of going swimming without supervision. Parents may occasionally have to help them keep a sensible balance between acknowledging the fact of their epilepsy and not letting it limit their life or activities unnecessarily.

Finally, if your life is a constant battle with a teenager who seems to you to be rebellious to the point of madness about his or her own well-being, remember that, as with every other adolescent, there is every chance they will eventually grow up and grow out of it.

COSMETIC EFFECTS OF MEDICATION

Refusal to comply with their drug regime may not be just an act of teenage rebellion, but based on a perfectly sound reason. Some young people, especially teenage girls, refuse to take their medication because as well as controlling seizures, some anti-epileptic drugs do, unfortunately, have undesirable cosmetic side-effects. Teenagers may have to suffer unwanted hairiness or hair loss, coarsening of the skin or excessive weight gain. Phenytoin is one of the worst culprits as regards spots and skin quality and sodium valproate may cause hair loss and weight gain.

Side-effects like these deal a blow to anybody's self-esteem, but for the teenager, for whom appearances count so much and who tend to be intensely self-conscious even at the best of times, they are especially hard to bear. Any teenager whose life is being made miserable by the cosmetic side-effects of medication should talk to their doctor about the possibility of changing drugs, even if their seizures are well controlled. It may be one of those situations where a slight increase in seizures is worth risking for the sake of the teenager's psychological well-being.

THE LURE OF THE DRIVING LICENCE

For many teenagers, the ability to drive is a hallmark of adulthood and a passport to independence. Unless the teenager's epilepsy is well controlled, he or she will be unable to obtain a driving licence (see p.136). So this is a carrot parents may find it valuable to dangle in front of the nose of the teenager with epilepsy who will not comply with their drug regime, or is reluctant to keep up regular clinic visits.

Recreational (street) drugs

Adolescence is a time of experimentation, and some adolescents are going to experiment with drugs, particularly in their middle or late teens. All parents worry about the drug culture that their child might become involved in, but my experience is that teenagers who have had epilepsy throughout their childhood are probably less likely than many of their peers to experiment with recreational drugs, perhaps because they are more 'drug-wise'. They have been brought up with a strict drug regime; they are used to using drugs therapeutically, and may be much more aware than most teenagers of the dangers of drug abuse.

Of those adolescents who do experiment with drugs, most will obtain them from friends and very few will have access to heroin, crack or cocaine. Marijuana (cannabis) is by far the most commonly-used drug amongst teenagers.

For their own safety teenagers need to be well informed about drugs and teenagers with epilepsy need to know the special risks they may be running if they experiment with drugs. Some recreational drugs may interact with anticonvulsant medication and some, particularly alcohol and cocaine, are themselves associated with seizures.

ALCOHOL

Teenage drinking is on the increase. An American study of high-school seniors in 1986 found that 91 per cent had tried alcohol, 65 per cent had consumed it within the past month, and 5 per cent drank alcohol daily. About 10 per cent of American high-school and university teenagers have been found to be 'heavy drinkers'. Neither is there as much difference as there used to be between the drinking habits of girls and boys, though girls are still less likely to drink regularly and heavily.

These are American figures, but all the evidence is that British teenagers are no different. Alcohol abuse is associated with poor seizure control (see pp.122–4), and the teenager with epilepsy must be told the risks of drinking, and taught that if they spend an evening in the pub with their friends, they can not match them drink for drink without being likely to have seizures the morning after. It is worth drawing their attention to low-alcohol beers and wines, while also making sure that they understand that whatever they drink they should try to keep their total fluid intake low so that they do not run the risk of a water load induced seizure (see p.122).

MARIJUANA

After alcohol and tobacco, marijuana is probably the recreational drug most often used by teenagers. Marijuana induces euphoria, heightened perceptions and a sense of relaxation at low doses. High doses have more complex effects, including fear, distortions of body image and disorientation. Marijuana also affects co-ordination, as do many antiepileptic drugs; if they are taken together the toxic effects on co-ordination and balance are likely to be greatly increased.

Some reports suggest that marijuana may reduce seizures, others that it may increase them. In fact, because the amounts used and the purity and type of the drug vary so widely it is difficult to come to any clear conclusions. There is no real evidence that it has any specific adverse effect when used by people with epilepsy. However, the heavy marijuana user may tend to be less compliant about taking his or her drugs. There is also a tendency for sleep cycles to be disturbed in heavy marijuana use, and both these factors may mean that a person's epilepsy becomes less well controlled.

AMPHETAMINES
(Common names: uppers, speed, pep pills, sulphate, blues, black bombers, purple hearts)

Amphetamines are stimulants, reasonably cheap and easy to get hold of, and usually taken to keep the user awake throughout an all-night party (or, a less credible scenario, to enable them to stay awake and revise for an exam). Amphetamines also reduce appetite.

Amphetamines used to be prescribed with anticonvulsant medication to counteract the drowsy side-effects although this is seldom done now. Amphetamines themselves probably do not cause seizures, but the chaotic life style they induce, with irregular meals and lack of sleep, may well do so.

ECSTASY

Ecstasy is the street name of a widely available amphetamine-like drug. As with amphetamines, it is largely a 'party' drug, keeping the user lively and happy so that they can sustain a party mood for hours without flagging. Many youngsters take it without any apparent ill-effects; others react badly, and some have died. This unpredictability makes it a dangerous drug for anyone; for the teenager with epilepsy it has special risks. Like amphetamines, its use is associated with disrupted sleep and skipped meals. Teenagers who take ecstasy become so lively and hyperactive that they often become dehydrated, which seems to increase the risks from the drug. To avoid dehydration they need to drink a lot (of water, not alcohol) and for someone with epilepsy drinking might itself produce a water overload and trigger off a seizure.

HEROIN
(Common names: H, smack, scag, horse, blow)

Heroin is a powerful drug causing both physical and psychological dependence. The first time it is taken it usually only causes nausea and vomiting. Only after it has been taken a few times is the 'rush' – a brief but intense feeling of pleasure and euphoria – experienced. The rush is followed by a feeling of calm and peace. Heroin can be dissolved in water and injected beneath the skin, into a muscle, or directly into a vein. Usually, however, it is smoked (called 'chasing the dragon') or sniffed, and taken this way the dangers of overdose and infection are reduced and the effects are less powerful.

Pure heroin does not cause seizures in ordinary doses (though it may do so in small children), neither does withdrawal of the drug cause seizures. The real danger (of which anyone who takes heroin, whether or not they have epilepsy, should be aware) is that most 'street heroin' is unlikely to be pure. Often it is mixed with substances like strychnine and other drugs which may well cause seizures.

COCAINE
(Common names: coke, snow, crack)

Cocaine is probably the most dangerous street drug for anyone who has epilepsy. It is a stimulant drug with effects very similar to amphetamines and is a potent seizure precipitant. Even people who do not have epilepsy may fit the first time they take cocaine. If you have epilepsy, the risks of having a seizure are very much greater.

Advice on future employment

One of the problems faced by adolescents with epilepsy is the difficulty of getting the right sort of job or, indeed, any job at all. Teenagers with epilepsy need help to prepare them for their search for employment. To begin with, they need realistic expectations. There are jobs which a diagnosis of epilepsy precludes (see pp.139–42). But more positively, proper assessment of their abilities and interests will help them decide what kind of job is likely to be appropriate.

Poor seizure control may be one limiting factor for the teenager who is looking for work, but it is by no means the only, or even the most important one. Medication may slow them down, for example. Often psychological factors (the teenager's poor self-image or lack of motivation, the fact that they lack self-confidence or still feel very dependent on their parents) may make them perform badly in job interviews and, when they do get a job, make it hard for them to cope when under stress.

A teenager who is having difficulty in finding work needs to be helped both to see him or herself in a different light, and to present him or herself to others more favourably. Parents can help by encouraging their child to be as independent as possible, and by boosting their self-esteem in any way they can, but it may be a good idea to get professional counselling as well.

Sexuality

SEXUAL DEVELOPMENT

In girls, some antiepileptic drugs may temporarily delay the onset of periods. A boy's sexual development is not usually affected. However, teenagers who have taken anticonvulsants since they were small children may not be quite as tall as their friends of the same age who do not have epilepsy.

SEX DRIVE

Children whose seizures continue into adolescence and who take anticonvulsants during this time are often said to have a lower sex drive as adults. This seems to be more true for boys than for girls. Certainly boys who have grown up with seizures during puberty are less likely to marry than girls who had epilepsy during adolescence. This statistic is probably at least partly because they do not have the sexual drive to go out and find a partner. It may be that some anticonvulsants have a direct effect on the testes, reducing the levels of the male sex hormone testosterone which is responsible for the sexual drive (see pp.43–58).

CONTRACEPTION

The oral contraceptive pill is a popular choice for adolescents. However, some anti-epileptic drugs – barbiturates, carbamazepine, phenytoin and ethosuximide – make the liver break down the pill more quickly so that it is less effective as a contraceptive (see p.190). This fact does not mean that the pill can not be prescribed, only that a higher dose may be needed if it is to be effective. This higher dose will not affect your health in any way.

For young people who are likely to have sex only irregularly, an alternative method may be a better solution. Other types of contraceptive (the condom, for example) are very effective if used properly. Although the condom is traditionally a 'male method', safer sex education has made it equally acceptable for a woman to carry condoms, and to insist on their use.

11

When Epilepsy Becomes A Handicap

Nearly everyone who has epilepsy lives a normal, ordinary life, with a family and a job. Only a very few are so disabled by their seizures that they can not have an independent existence. And for many of these people the real cause of their disability is usually not the epilepsy itself, but the fact that the brain damage which is responsible for their seizures is severe enough to cause learning disabilities too. However, despite even their double handicap, people with both epilepsy and brain damage can still lead a fulfilled life.

AN ORDINARY LIFE

The move away from institutional care towards community-based care has meant that many people with special needs can now look forward to living an ordinary life within their local community. Small group homes, run by local authorities or housing associations aim to give people with learning disabilities as much support as they need whilst at the same time encouraging their independence and self-development. Staffing levels and levels of support will depend on an individual resident's needs. This may range from round-the-clock care with night staff, to daily visits from carers. In addition, local Community

Learning Disability Teams often work closely with staff and residents from the homes, to help sort out any problems that arise.

One of the difficulties which people with epilepsy have to overcome is other people's tendency to over-protect them and so make them more dependent. People with learning disabilities need to learn to become as independent as possible, and with help many can take the basic steps towards achieving at least a measure of self-reliance. When someone has severe learning disabilities, they may need to learn how to make simple choices, how to dress or wash themselves, or how to take part in some other aspect of self care. Those with less severe learning disabilities may be able to reach a level of self-reliance that allows them to have an independent life in a home of their own. Everyone, whatever their level of disability, has the potential to achieve greater independence.

Children with learning disabilities

The policy of education authorities is that as many children with epilepsy as possible should go to normal, mainstream schools, and about 60 per cent of adolescents with epilepsy are in regular classrooms attending normal schools. However, learning disabilities are more common amongst teenagers with epilepsy. For those who are most severely disabled a normal school may not be possible, and there are three special schools for children with severe epilepsy, including those with learning disabilities (see Appendix). These schools are run like normal boarding schools. However, because it is the policy of many education authorities not to send children out of the area if they believe the child's educational needs can be met within it, parents who want to send their child to one of these schools may have difficulty in obtaining the necessary funding.

HELP AVAILABLE

If your child has both learning disabilities and epilepsy, you need help, not only to make sure that your child's needs are met, but so that you yourself get support, someone to talk to who knows about the strain this can put on a family and will be able to advise you if problems arise.

Your GP will put you in touch with the appropriate team of professionals who will assess your child's needs and give you specialist support and help at home. Their job is also to liaise with schools, or with a young person's place of work, look at any problems there and help work out a solution.

The kind of support provided varies from region to region. In some areas, children with disabilities are catered for within the normal child services. In other areas these children may be seen by a specialist Child Development Team, and in others by the Community Learning Disabilities Team. Most teams consist of professionals from both Health and Social Services, which usually ensures that there is co-ordination between the various aspects of care or help that are needed. In general, health professionals are responsible for ensuring that someone's health needs (both physical and mental) are met. Social service staff are responsible for looking at their housing, financial, employment and social support needs, and in some areas may have responsibility for co-ordinating a package of care between the various agencies. The local education authority is responsible for meeting a child's educational needs. More often than not, you may well find yourself having to deal with several different professionals or agencies to get all the help that you need.

SPECIAL PROBLEMS

The combination of epilepsy and brain damage may cause special problems. If you have a child with learning disabilities as well as epilepsy, there are several points of which you should be aware.

- Someone who has brain damage may respond differently to drugs. The side-effects of drugs may be stronger, and they may be more likely to cause difficult or abnormal behaviour.
- After a seizure someone with brain damage may be more profoundly affected than other people. It may take them longer (perhaps a matter of days rather than hours) to get back to normal.
- People with learning disabilities sometimes have very severe epilepsy and it is important for them to wear protective headgear to protect them if they fall. This headgear is usually something very like a motorcycle helmet. When a child has to wear protective headgear it is yet another way of being made to feel different from other children. Be sensitive to the child's feelings; there are some nicely-designed headpieces on the market which may make them feel less conspicuous. One alternative version is available from the David Lewis Centre for Epilepsy which has designed a protective headpiece in the form of a wig with hair attached to a fibreglass protective base. It is both less cumbersome and less conspicuous than the traditional helmet.
- Just because a child has learning disabilities it does not mean that their epilepsy should not be properly investigated. Never let anyone tell you that it is 'not worth' referring a child for special investigations: EEG, an MRI scan or psychometry. As a parent you will probably want to know the cause of your child's epilepsy even if that information does not make any difference to the course of the condition.
- In the same way, learning disabilities should not prevent a child from being considered for epilepsy surgery, though they may not be suitable if they have generalized brain damage. If seizures arise from a specific focus surgery may

cure the epilepsy, though it can not cure the learning disabilities. It may, however, prevent the learning disabilities from getting worse, because people who have very frequent and severe seizures do often suffer some mental deterioration.

COPING WITH AGGRESSION

Aggression is not characteristic of epilepsy, but it is, quite often, a by-product of brain damage. Drugs may also contribute to aggressive behaviour. Any anticonvulsant can occasionally cause aggression, but the biggest culprits are the sedative drugs, myselin and phenobarbitone. Sometimes phenytoin has the same effect, as does, less often, sodium valproate.

So it is not surprising that children who are brain damaged and often taking more than one anticonvulsant drug are sometimes irritable and aggressive; often their behaviour is problematic in other ways too. However, when a child is very aggressive or badly behaved, there are very often other causes besides drugs.

Difficult behaviour of any kind arouses very strong emotions in parents. Inevitably your own emotions are going to affect the way you respond to the child; the chances are that you will feel angry, and if you do you are likely to respond angrily. This reaction is understandable, but unfortunately a negative response to difficult behaviour often has the effect of reinforcing it and making it worse.

How to respond

How you respond to someone who seems to be behaving 'badly' depends very much on *why* you think they are behaving this way. If you think that the child could, if they wanted to, control their behaviour, that it is simply part of their personality, or a direct attempt to manipulate you, then you are much more likely to be angry with them than if you saw the behaviour as something that is a by-product of their disability, and therefore largely outside their control. In this latter case you would know the child could not help what it was doing, and you would be more likely to be sympathetic. You would feel pity rather than anger, and you would probably be more tolerant and respond much more positively to them.

If you can analyse your child's behaviour quite closely, so that you can see what has led up to it and what its consequences are, you may understand it better (keeping an ABC chart in the way suggested on pp.97–100 is one way to do this). Sometimes, for example, a child uses 'bad' or aggressive behaviour as a way of communicating. The child may feel emotions – 'I'm frightened,' or 'I've had enough' – but may not have the words to express them. Aggression may be the only way they can 'say' what they feel. And if at the same time you examine your own beliefs about the causes underlying the child's behaviour, you may understand your own emotions and perhaps feel better able to deal with them and to respond to your child in a different way. Sometimes, for example, parents are comforted by believing that their child has some control over his or her behaviour; they themselves need not then feel so responsible and guilty about it.

If your child's behaviour is a problem, ask for help from the specialist professionals in either the Child Development Team or the Community Team for Learning Disabilities. Many areas have special intensive support teams who will work either with the family or with the school, to help manage and reduce aggression or other problems. Drug treatment is very seldom the answer, though sometimes it can help modify aggressive behaviour.

It is also worth bearing in mind that psychiatric illnesses such as depression or schizophrenia may show themselves quite differently in someone who has severe learning disabilities. Someone who is depressed, for example, may not necessarily appear to be sad; instead their behaviour may deteriorate quite markedly.

LOOKING TO THE FUTURE

What will happen to our child when we are gone? Any parent whose child has profound difficulties worries about the future and has probably asked themselves this question. It is an anxiety

178

that has to be faced and the best insurance policy for your child's future is for you to try and ensure that they achieve a degree of independence while you are alive. You might aim, for example, to get them established in a group home when they become adult.

However, in some regions this will be easier than in others. It will depend on the extent of accommodation available and the state of social service funding. Social services departments or your local Community Learning Disabilities Team are the first people to approach. They will know what facilities are available in your area, including houses run by housing associations and privately run homes. They will also help to assess whether the accommodation will meet the needs of your child. In addition, social services hold the purse strings, and any application, whether to a privately run home or to a home run by a housing association will need funding agreement by your local social services department.

Letting your child go

Even if you are lucky enough to find just the right home for your child, where they will be competently cared for and have just the right mixture of companionship, care and independence, your own feelings about the move will probably be mixed. Most parents in this situation feel a mixture of guilt ('We should be able to continue to look after our own child; it's our job'), as well as a very natural sense of relief. They may feel anxiety ('Will anyone else be able to take care of our child as well as we can?'), and huge personal loss. Looking after your child has probably taken up a large part of your life; it has given you a role and a purpose and it may take you some time to come to terms with this dual loss. But however hard it is for you, independence has to be the best decision you can make for your child.

TREATMENT OPTIONS FOR SEVERE EPILEPSY

When a child's epilepsy is very severe, a doctor may pile on drug after drug, in a desperate attempt to get better seizure control.

However, after a certain point there is often little benefit to the child in this course of action. Obviously when a child has severe epilepsy the doctor has to aim to reduce the frequency of seizures. But a balance also has to be struck; prescribing ever more anticonvulsants may simply make the child increasingly slow and drowsy without having much extra effect on seizures. If your child seems to be very over-drugged, it may be better to talk to your doctor about the possibility of cutting down the number of different medications they are taking so that they become brighter and more alert, even though that means accepting that their seizure frequency will not be reduced any further.

A few children have intractable epilepsy combined with very severe physical disability, for example a hemiplegia (paralysis of one side of their body). They may be able to walk, but otherwise have little useful function on one side of their brain. The risk for these children is that the severe, unremitting seizures arising in the damaged side of the brain may gradually damage the other, 'good' side of the brain, so that they no longer acquire any further skills and may actually deteriorate, losing those skills they already have. For these few children the operation of hemispherectomy, to remove the damaged half of the brain (see p.71) is worth considering.

Hemispherectomy is only an option if damage is extensive but confined to one side of the brain. But for these few children it can greatly improve the quality of life. They have fewer seizures, need fewer drugs, and become brighter, more responsive and sometimes less aggressive and better behaved too. Parents often say they notice this change in behaviour almost immediately after the operation.

Some rare disabling conditions

LENNOX GASTAUT SYNDROME

A few of the children who are most severely disabled with epilepsy suffer from a rare condition, Lennox Gastaut syndrome. These children have very severe learning disabilities, it is impossible to control their seizures with drugs, and their condition gradually deteriorates. A drug called felbamate can give some seizure control, but the drug itself has some dangerous side-effects and is only used in special circumstances.

LANDAU KLEFFNE

Landau Kleffne is a very rare syndrome in which a child develops seizures, until, at the age of five, their speech starts to regress and they may stop speaking. Although it is extremely rare and affects only a very few children, Landau Kleffne is worth mentioning simply because if it is diagnosed early the condition is reversible and an operation can be done to stop the damage to speech. If the child is not referred to a specialist in time, their speech may be permanently damaged.

RASMUSSEN'S SYNDROME

In rare cases, a child may develop severe epilepsy which seems to come from one side of the brain. They may then start to lose some mental skills and, more important, their movement and coordination of the side of the body opposite to the affected side of the brain, may start to deteriorate slowly. The child therefore becomes increasingly handicapped. At this stage, an MRI scan may show that half the brain has started to atrophy. In severe cases, the treatment is hemispherectomy. This degeneration of one half of the brain is known as Rasmussens encephalitis (or Rasmussen's syndrome), and it is thought to be caused by a virus which attacks one half of the brain, but not the other.

Employment opportunities

FINDING A JOB

If you have been out of work for some time and have difficulty finding a job you can seek help from one of the Manpower Service Commission's disablement resettlement officers (DROs). It may be that as a first step to helping you find a job, they will suggest that you apply (with their help) for a stay at one of the MSC's rehabilitation centres, where you will be helped to establish a working routine and given advice about future employment. The next step may be to join a Training Opportunities course which will equip you with a special skill.

While you are doing these courses you will be given a tax-free living allowance, and your National Insurance record will be kept up to date by giving a credit of contributions.

REGISTERING AS DISABLED

Every handicapped person has to decide whether there is any advantage in being registered as a disabled person, or whether this might actually put off a prospective employer. There are advantages in being registered as disabled, and the more severely you are handicapped, the greater these advantages are likely to be. The registered disabled person can apply for sheltered employment and assistance with taxi fares to work if they are too severely handicapped to use public transport or drive

WHEN EPILEPSY BECOMES A HANDICAP

themselves, for example. Employers of over 20 people are obliged by law to employ a quota of three per cent disabled people.

SHELTERED EMPLOYMENT

The DRO can help people who are too disabled to manage an ordinary job to find a job in sheltered employment. These jobs are available either through a government-sponsored company which provides work for nearly 8,000 people, or in a workshop run by a local authority or voluntary organization. Some local authorities employ people with epilepsy to work in parks and gardens; anyone doing such a job will be paid the full rate for it.

chapter twelve

Sex, Pregnancy and Epilepsy

E veryone has some kind of sexual problem at some time in their life, and people with epilepsy are no exception. If you have epilepsy you are almost bound to have to deal with, at some time or another, the same sexual problems that most people occasionally encounter. Sex is not always perfect. Many men have erection problems, many women find it difficult to reach orgasm. People vary very much in their need for sex, their interest in it, and even in their enjoyment of it.

In addition to these 'normal' problems which everyone has, people who have epilepsy may also have sexual anxieties and occasionally problems which are related to their epilepsy. Many, perhaps most, of the special sexual problems of people with epilepsy are a by-product of anticonvulsant medication. But most of these problems can be solved. Epilepsy need not stop you starting a family, or affect your chances of marriage or of having normal sexual relationships.

Marriage

Even now there are parts of the world where misconceptions about epilepsy are still widespread. It is often assumed that epilepsy is entirely an inherited disease, and there may also be fears and taboos surrounding it. In these cultures, especially if arranged marriages are the norm, the marriage prospects of a woman with epilepsy are slim. If she is already married when she develops epilepsy, she may have to be returned to her family.

But these are special cases. In the West a woman with epilepsy has no need to worry about her chances of marriage. They are now exactly the same as those of a woman who does not have epilepsy.

The news is not so good for men. Most studies have shown that men who have epilepsy seem to be less likely to marry than men who do not have the condition, and much less likely to marry than women who have epilepsy. It is difficult to pin-point the reason for this. One explanation is that even now, when sexual roles in society are less rigid than they used to be, men still tend to take the initiative in sexual relationships. It may be that men who are taking anticonvulsant drugs may be less likely to make the first move in a relationship. One of the side-effects of these drugs (see pp.43–58) is a reduction in sexual drive and interest.

And yet even if sex is not such a powerful driving force for these men, it is still surprising that many of them do not marry. Anticonvulsants may reduce the desire for sex; they do not make the need for a loving relationship any less. Indeed, one research study found that men who have epilepsy attach even more importance to having a partner or being married than do women with epilepsy.

If you want to get married, but have not yet managed to make the right kind of relationship, it might be worth your while having counselling to help you gain the sexual confidence to make the first approach. Ask your GP or the local mental health services to refer you for sexual counselling.

You can also take steps to help yourself, the first one being to get involved in some activity which will help you meet more people. An evening class or some voluntary work could be a start, or joining an epilepsy support group if you do not already belong to one. When you do meet someone you like, do not feel you have to rush things, but get to know them and feel comfortable with them as a friend before you become involved in a sexual relationship.

Sexual side-effects of epilepsy

LACK OF SEXUAL INTEREST

The most common sexual side-effect of epilepsy is simply lack of interest. In men, the sex hormone, testosterone, is produced in the testes. If the levels of testosterone are low, sex drive and sexual interest are lowered too, and it may be more difficult to get an erection. Some anticonvulsant drugs have a direct effect on the testes and reduce the amount of testosterone they produce. Other drugs have an indirect effect on testosterone levels by altering liver function. When the liver has to work harder, one result is an increase in the blood level of a protein which 'binds' to testosterone, so there is less free 'working' testosterone circulating in the blood. In this case the testes are working quite normally, but they cannot increase their production of sex hormone enough to compensate for this extra binding.

People who lack sexual interest will have sex less often than many other people, but this is not to say they have a problem. There are plenty of people in the general population who have sex seldom or even never, and who are perfectly happy with things as they are. It can become a problem if you are worried that you are missing out on a side of life that you would like to experience. If you have a partner it may cause difficulties if they are more interested in sex than you are. Lack of interest may lead to other problems too: a man may have difficulty getting an erection, for example, or a woman finds she seldom feels sexually aroused or reaches orgasm.

If your lack of interest in sex worries you, it may be worth asking your doctor if you can have tests to check your level of testosterone. Some doctors, though not all, recommend testosterone replacement therapy to men who are worried about a lack of sexual interest and whose testosterone level is low. It is not a treatment much used at the moment, but it is worth asking your doctor about it if you have this problem.

Although lack of interest in sex is nearly always a result of anticonvulsant drugs, there is some suggestion that a few men who have very frequent seizures during adolescence have a low sexual drive and reduced sexual interest when they become adults, even though they have normal levels of sex hormones.

FEAR OF SEIZURES DURING SEX

Perhaps the main sexual anxiety of those people with epilepsy who have a sexual partner is that they will have a seizure during intercourse. There is the fear of looking unattractive, putting their partner off or possibly even ruining the relationship. It is an understandable fear and yet it is also an unrealistic one. You are in fact no more likely to have a seizure during sex than at any other time of the day or night. The odds against it happening are high, so there is really no need for you to feel apprehensive about it. You certainly should not let the idea of it happening put you off sex or make you reluctant to have intercourse. It is also very rare indeed for sexual activity to be a *specific* trigger for seizures; I have never come across anyone who has experienced this condition, and only a very few such cases have ever been reported.

A few women always find it hard to 'let go' during sex; they fear the loss of control which sex involves, and this often prevents them reaching orgasm. It is possible that for some women this anxiety lies at the heart of their fear of seizures during sex; it is part of a general reluctance to 'let go' during sex rather than a specific fear of seizure. If you think these feelings may be playing a part in your fears, psychosexual counselling from a qualified therapist might help you resolve them.

Women and epilepsy

Women whose epilepsy started when they were children very often find that when they reach puberty the nature of their epilepsy changes. About two-thirds of women experience some sort of change. Usually there is an increase in seizure frequency, or a new type of seizure develops. But in about a third of cases the change is positive; seizure frequency decreases and seizures may even stop altogether. As a general rule, absence seizures tend to become less frequent or to stop. The chances of a woman's epilepsy getting worse at puberty are greater if she reaches puberty later than average, or if her epilepsy started early in childhood, or if she has an abnormal EEG and has previously had a great many generalized tonic clonic seizures.

MENSTRUATION AND EPILEPSY

Does epilepsy affect periods?
It is very unusual for a woman's periods to be affected if she develops epilepsy. However, a few women have seizures which affect the part of the brain that regulates the menstrual cycle, and in this case they may be more likely than other women to have menstrual problems such as irregular periods. In addition, some

anti-epileptic drugs, particularly sodium valproate (Epilim) affect the menstrual cycle.

Do periods affect epilepsy?
Nearly everyone who has epilepsy discovers that the frequency of their seizures varies. There will be times when you seem to have more seizures than at others. So it is not surprising that quite often a woman notices that she seems to have more seizures around the time of her period. However, if you keep a seizure diary you will probably find that this does not happen every month. Seizures are nearly always more irregular and unpredictable than this.

Catamenial epilepsy
A few women (probably less than 10 per cent of all women with epilepsy) *do* have what is called catamenial epilepsy – a type of epilepsy in which every month there is a regular and definite increase in seizure frequency around menstruation. Often they start to have regular, recurrent 'bad patches' of seizures just before they reach puberty. When their periods start it is clear that they have catamenial epilepsy.

Catamenial epilepsy is probably somehow related to the relative levels of the hormones oestrogen and progesterone which are produced during the menstrual cycle, though it is difficult to find a clear relationship. The normal pattern is that during the first half of the menstrual cycle, oestrogen is the main hormone produced. During the second half of the cycle both oestrogen and progesterone are produced. Oestrogen is known to have a seizure-provoking effect, while progesterone is an anticonvulsant and tends to protect against seizures.

But even if hormones play a part, they cannot provide a complete explanation, because there does not seem to be any noticeable difference in the hormonal changes between women who have catamenial epilepsy and those whose epilepsy is no worse at the time of their periods. Another explanation is that pre-menstrual tension may play a part, and that women with catamenial epilepsy are more likely to suffer PMT. Stress and anxiety are known to precipitate seizures and the mood changes of PMT may have something to do with their seizure increase at that time. At the moment, however, this is only a theory.

EPILEPSY AND FERTILITY

Another worry many women have is that epilepsy may affect their ability to conceive. Fertility rates are slightly reduced in both men and women with epilepsy. Women may find it more difficult to become pregnant if seizures affect the part of the brain that regulates the menstrual cycle and they experience irregular periods, or if they are taking anticonvulsants which affect the menstrual cycle. Yet although you may take a little longer to become pregnant, these factors will not stop you conceiving. If after a year of trying you are still not pregnant, talk to your doctor. Modern methods of fertility treatment should solve the problem.

EPILEPSY AND CONTRACEPTION

Hormonal contraception ('The Pill')
Hormonal contraception is a safe and very effective form of birth control. It can be taken orally, in the form of the combined pill (which contains two hormones, oestrogen and progesterone) or the progesterone-only 'mini-pill'. It can also be given as a slowly absorbed (depot) injection or an implant under the skin. These two methods have the advantages that the implant or injection lasts several weeks, and you do not have to remember to take a pill every day.

Because it is so effective, hormonal contraception, usually in the form of the Pill, is the method of first choice for many women. However, if you have epilepsy, you need to discuss its pros and cons with your doctor before you decide it is the right method for you.

If you are taking sodium valproate, vigabatrin, lamotrigine, gabapentin, clobazam, clonazepam or ethosuximide, there is no problem and you can take the oral contraceptives, or use contraceptive injections or implants, in the normal way. However, a few widely-used anticonvulsants (phenytoin, phenobarbitone, carbamazepine, and primidone) make the liver break down the hormones in these contraceptive preparations more rapidly, reducing their effectiveness. The sign that the contraceptive effect of the pill has failed is that you get 'breakthrough' bleeding.

You are not prevented from using hormonal contraception if you are taking any of these latter drugs, but for them to be effective you may need to take a higher than usual dose of the oral contraceptive, or receive more frequent injections or implants. The dose of the Pill, for example, may need to be increased two or three times until you have a cycle with no breakthrough bleeding. Until you have a cycle without breakthrough bleeding you will need to use a condom or some other form of contraception.

The larger dose of the contraceptive will not have any more side-effects than the normal one, because the excess hormone is being broken down and disposed of by the liver.

A few women with epilepsy find that the Pill makes their epilepsy worse. But it is more likely that going on the Pill will reduce your seizure frequency by helping to reduce pre-menstrual seizures. Some women therefore decide to take the pill continually on a 28 day cycle without the usual seven days' break.

If it is to be effective, the pill has to be taken regularly, every day and at the same time every day. Remembering to take it may be a problem if you have frequent seizures. If you want a hormonal method of contraception, but do not feel that you can rely on your memory to take the Pill regularly, contraceptive injections or implants may be a better solution. These are hormones with a long-term effect and are either given by injection or implanted beneath the skin. This must be done by a doctor or specially-trained family planning nurse.

Emergency contraception
Emergency contraception used to be known as the 'morning after' pill, but in fact it need not be taken the morning after

unprotected intercourse. Ideally, it should be taken within 3 days (72 hours) of having sex. However, it may even work if taken within five days; sperm can survive for a couple of days, and so it is always possible that you may have ovulated and conceived two days after having sex. The pill consists of two hormonal pills taken immediately, and another two taken 12 hours later. You can use emergency contraception if you are taking anticonvulsant medication, but, depending on the drug you are taking, you may need a slightly larger dose. If you tell the doctor who gives it to you that you have epilepsy, and what drugs you are on, your anticonvulsant medication can be taken into account.

MENOPAUSE

The menopause is often another time of seizure change though, as ever, epilepsy is so unpredictable that it is difficult to say which direction the change will take. Seizures may increase or decrease in frequency, go into remission, recur if they have been in remission or there may be no change at all. And a few women who have never had seizures before in their lives may start to have them at the menopause, though no one knows the reason for this.

If your seizures have always been related to your periods they will probably improve during the menopause. You can also feel optimistic about improvement if your seizures began late in life and have always been infrequent. However, there is some evidence that in women who have an earlier than average menopause seizure frequency tends to remain unchanged, or to increase.

EPILEPSY AND HRT

One of the inevitable results of old age is that bones grow less dense and more brittle (a condition called osteoporosis). Until women reach the menopause, oestrogen gives some protection against thinning of the bones, and many doctors advise women to have hormone replacement therapy (HRT) to prevent osteoporosis. This is especially important for women who have a family history of osteoporosis. It is also very important for women with epilepsy, because anticonvulsant drugs, particularly phenytoin, tend to cause calcium deficiency and increase the risk of brittle bones.

HRT contains the same hormones as the contraceptive pill, and so you may need to take a higher dose than normal to be effective if you are taking phenytoin, phenobarbitone, carbamazepine, or primidone (see Hormonal contraceptives, p.190). In a few women HRT increases seizure frequency, though if you have this problem it may be possible for you to find a different form of HRT which does not have this effect.

Pregnancy

Mary and her husband felt it was time they started a family. Only one thing made them hesitate – Mary's epilepsy. The drug she had to take to control her generalized seizures was sodium valproate and she knew there was a chance that this might damage her baby.

So before trying to get pregnant, they came to see me. 'I've thought about it very carefully, and I'd like to come off drugs altogether while I'm pregnant,' Mary told me firmly. 'I know I'm risking having seizures, but I'm not worried about that. I think it's more important not to risk damaging my baby. And I know perfectly well that there's no drug you can give me which is guaranteed to be safe during pregnancy.'

I knew very well how Mary felt. But I had to tell her that it wasn't quite as simple as that. If Mary did have her usual generalized seizure, this too would put her baby at risk, because during the seizure the baby might be deprived of oxygen. So I suggested a third option, which was to change Mary's anti-convulsant drug from sodium valproate to Tegretol, a drug which was safer for pregnant women to take. However, this change would mean postponing the pregnancy for another few months, to make sure that the new drug suited Mary and controlled her seizures.

Three months later, her seizures well controlled with Tegretol, Mary became pregnant. And nine months after that, their baby was born – an eight and a half pound, perfectly healthy, baby boy.

If you have epilepsy and want to become pregnant, you need to think ahead, and discuss your plans with your doctor well in advance. Anticonvulsant drugs can sometimes damage the developing foetus, and your doctor will want to make sure that you are taking the safest possible drug before you try to conceive. If he or she feels it is appropriate, they may suggest that you change to another anticonvulsant. Unfortunately no anti-epileptic drug is entirely safe in pregnancy, but carbamazepine (Tegretol) is thought to be the least harmful. The risk is higher if you are taking more than one antiepileptic drug.

The risk of having a baby with a birth defect may also be higher if there is a history of birth defects in the family of either parent. Genetic counselling before you embark on the pregnancy will help you assess what the risk is in your particular case.

No one specific abnormality is associated with antiepileptic drugs, but the commonest problems are:

- Cleft lip and/or palate and congenital heart defects (associated with phenytoin);
- Spina bifida, malformation of the penis, 'webbed' fingers or toes (sodium valproate);
- Possibly reduced birth weight and slow development (carbamazepine);
- Malformations of the face, for example eyes which are set too wide apart (commonly phenytoin).

So, if *no* anticonvulsant is entirely safe, you may well feel like asking your doctor if you can discontinue your drugs entirely during your pregnancy. There are two arguments against this course of action. The first thing to realize is that although there is a risk in taking anticonvulsants, it is still only a very small one. In the population as a whole, two or three babies in every hundred are born with some birth defect. Amongst babies born to women with epilepsy who are taking anticonvulsants the rate of birth defects is four to six in every hundred babies. The risk is increased, but it is still not a large risk.

Second, until very recently it was generally accepted that, when a woman had seizures during pregnancy, her baby was at risk because it might be deprived of oxygen during a seizure, particularly if she went into *status epilepticus*. More recent evidence suggests that this may not be so, though doctores are not yet certain. What is certain, however, is that the woman herself runs a risk if she stops taking anticonvulsants.

So the chances are that your doctor will probably advise you to carry on taking medication. In the end, though, you are the one who has to balance the risks and make the decision. If you do continue taking your drugs, try not to worry. Remember that, despite taking anticonvulsants, nearly all women with epilepsy have normal pregnancies and healthy babies.

All women are advised now to take folic acid for a month before they start trying to become pregnant, and to continue to take it for the first three months of pregnancy. Folic acid supplements have been found to reduce the risk of spina bifida and other nervous-system defects. It is especially important for women with epilepsy to take folic acid supplements, as some anticonvulsant drugs can reduce the levels of folic acid. Folic acid tablets can be bought over the counter without a prescription, and you should take one 0.4 mg tablet a day. Some doctors recommend that women who are taking carbamazepine or sodium valproate should take a higher dose of 4–5 mg daily. This same higher dose is also given to women who have previously given birth to a child with spina bifida.

You will probably also be asked to take vitamin K tablets for the last two weeks of pregnancy as some antiepileptic drugs cause vitamin K deficiency, which can produce a rare blood disorder.

In addition, your baby will be given a dose of vitamin K soon after birth, to protect against this disorder.

UNPLANNED PREGNANCY

If you did not plan to become pregnant but find that you are, without having had a chance to discuss changing your medication with your doctor, what should you do? Do not stop taking your drugs (this may lead to more seizures, which could also damage the baby) but see your doctor as soon as you can. He or she will be able to tell you how great a risk there is of you having a baby with some abnormality (the risks for most drugs are known). Clonazepam is one of the anticonvulsants with the highest risk of foetal abnormality, so if you are taking this drug, it is especially important to see your doctor straight away. Start taking folic acid tablets immediately (see p.195) and make sure you have appropriate screening tests for abnormalities of the baby (see below).

ANTENATAL SCREENING

Many birth defects can be detected by special screening tests during pregnancy. Most hospitals offer ultrasound scanning around 18 weeks and give a blood screening test around the 16th week of pregnancy to assess the risks of congenital disorder in the baby. Higher than normal levels of one chemical, AFP (Alpha Fetoprotein) can indicate a neural tube defect such as spina bifida.

The results of the test will be reported as 'screen positive' or 'screen negative'. But if you are told your test is positive, it does not necessarily mean that your baby has any abnormality. Screening tests can only assess risks. They are not diagnostic; they cannot confirm that a baby does or does not have spina bifida, only that there is a higher than average risk that it may. There are other reasons for a raised level of AFP; – it may simply be that your pregnancy is more advanced than was thought, for example. Most women who test screen positive go on to have perfectly healthy babies. However, a screen positive result does indicate that there is a need for further tests such as an ultrasound scan and possibly an amniocentesis, which can confirm whether or not there is any abnormality.

If it is found that your baby does have a serious defect, you can then decide whether to continue with the pregnancy.

ANXIETIES ABOUT PREGNANCY

Inheriting epilepsy
Inevitably, anyone with epilepsy who is thinking of starting a family is going to worry that their child might develop the condition too. So what is the likelihood that this might happen? The chances that anyone will develop epilepsy during their lifetime are about one in 200. If either you or your partner (but not both) have epilepsy, the chances of your child developing the condition are only about one in 40. If both parents have epilepsy the risk is higher. But even so, it is much more likely that your child will not develop epilepsy than that they will.

Seizures during pregnancy
Women with epilepsy are considered to have high-risk pregnancies, mostly because there is an increased risk of seizures during pregnancy, labour and delivery. About a quarter to a third of women have more seizures than usual during pregnancy, but some women have fewer. Unfortunately there is no way of predicting how any individual woman will react, whether she will have more or fewer seizures during her pregnancy. Neither does the course of one pregnancy make it any easier to predict what will happen in a second.

Doctors also have to take into account the slightly increased risks to the babies of women with epilepsy. Although these risks are small, they do exist. Babies of mothers with epilepsy are more likely to be born prematurely or to be of low birth weight, and rates of stillbirth are also slightly higher for these babies. Because of these risks it is not advisable for you to have a home birth. Your doctor will probably recommend that you have your baby in hospital.

Breastfeeding and baby care

Breastfeeding is best for your baby, and if you want to breastfeed, there is no reason why you should not do so. Even if you are taking anticonvulsant medication you can breastfeed quite safely. Although your drugs will pass into the breast milk, they will be in such small quantities that they do not affect the baby. The exceptions are phenobarbitone and diazepam, which may make the baby drowsy.

However, if lack of sleep is an important trigger factor for your seizures, it may be more practical for you to bottle feed, so that you can share the disturbed nights with your partner.

Safety precautions
Your epilepsy does not present any risk to your baby, except for the small one that he might be dropped if you have a fit while holding him. A few common-sense precautions are a good idea:

- Sit on floor cushions while feeding your baby;
- Wash and change the baby on a waterproof mat on the floor, rather than on a bed or high surface;
- **Do not bath your baby if you are alone.**

Immunization
Some parents who have epilepsy are reluctant to have their babies immunized, because they believe that some vaccines, particularly the whooping cough vaccine (included in the triple vaccine given to babies at two, three and four months and again as a booster at four to five years) may cause seizures.

If you think that your child is slightly more at risk of developing epilepsy than other children, because they may have inherited the tendency from you, it is understandable that you should want to do everything you can to avoid increasing that risk further. At the moment the weight of the medical evidence is that vaccination *is* safe for children, and that the real risks come from *not* vaccinating your children so that they are vulnerable to the disease. The current Department of Health guidelines are that even those children who have a close family relative with epilepsy should be immunized. However, this question is something that you should discuss with your doctor at the appropriate time, to make sure that you have the best and most up-to-date advice available.

13
POSTSCRIPT

When you, or your child, are given a diagnosis of epilepsy, it may seem as though your whole life has collapsed around you. It is a disorder that few people understand and about which most people have misconceptions. Everything you have ever read or heard about epilepsy, and the prejudices you have heard other people voice may combine to fuel your fears about the future.

It need not be like this. Never think of yourself (and discourage other people from thinking of you) as an 'epileptic'. Your seizures are epileptic; you are not. Even if seizures have to be part of your life for quite a long time to come, they will not necessarily be a large or important part of it. There is life after epilepsy and, even more important, there should be *quality* of life after epilepsy. Our hope is that this book will help you understand your epilepsy better, and so enable you to minimize its place in your life.

Absence seizure   A generalized seizure causing a brief loss of awareness that may look like day-dreaming. Associated with a characteristic EEG change of three spikes and waves (q.v.) per second. Seldom occurs after adolescence.

Acupuncture   A branch of Chinese medicine, in which special needles are inserted into channels (meridians) in the body along which the life force is said to flow. Some studies have shown that it can be effective in epilepsy; others doubt that it is.

Anticonvulsant   Drug used for treating seizures.

Aromatherapy   A therapy in which relaxation is induced by massaging the body with fragrant oils. Used as an alternative, behavioural treatment for epilepsy. The subject learns to associate the smell of the oil with whatever counter measure (q.v.) has been found to abort a seizure.

Aura   A feeling or sensation that is part of a partial seizure and occurs as it begins. The characteristics of the aura will depend on the part of the brain involved. Some seizures consist of the aura alone.

Behavioural treatment   Any method in which patients are taught how to modify their behaviour so as to reduce the frequency or severity of their seizures.

Biofeedback   A technique for reducing seizure frequency by learning to modify brain activity so as to produce an anti-convulsant effect.

Bourneville's disease   See Tuberous Sclerosis

Callostomy   An operation to separate the nerves connecting the two sides of the brain.

Complex partial seizure   A partial seizure (q.v.) which spreads out from its point of origin and affects consciousness.

Convulsion   Violent, involuntary muscular spasms which occur in a tonic clonic seizure. Often used as a synonym for seizure.

CT (Computerized Tomography)   A way of producing images of the structure of the brain by measuring the way X-rays are absorbed by the brain.

Counter measure   A piece of behaviour used at seizure onset either to inhibit the seizure completely, or to stop its spread.

Desensitization   A method which uses relaxation and imagery to help reduce anxiety about the idea of having a seizure.

Drop attack   A sudden very brief loss of consciousness and muscle tone, causing the person to drop suddenly to the ground.

Dysembryoplastic neuroepithelial tumour (DNT)   A benign, congenital lesion which causes epilepsy, usually in the temporal lobe.

Dysphasia   An inability to find the correct words.

Electrode   A small silver disk which is glued to the skull to record the small electrical currents of the brain during an EEG recording (q.v.).

Electroencephalogram   An electroencephalogram (EEG) records the electrical activity of the brain – the 'brain waves'. Abnormalities of electrical activity show up on the first EEG recording in about 75 per cent of people who have epilepsy.

EEG telemetry   See video monitoring

Epigastric aura   A feeling that arises in the stomach and moves up to the throat, usually accompanied by an intense sensation of fear. Often occurs at the beginning of a temporal lobe seizure.

Epilepsy   A tendency to have recurrent seizures. For the diagnosis to be made, two fits with no obvious cause must occur within two years.

Febrile convulsion A seizure caused by a high temperature. Febrile convulsions run in families and only affect children.

Fit Another word for seizure (q.v.).

Focal seizure The old term for partial seizure (q.v.).

Focus A small area of abnormal brain which gives rise to seizure activity.

Foramen ovale telemetry A temeletry EEG recording (q.v.) to record activity deep in the temporal lobe. Special wires are inserted through a hole in the skull (the foramen ovale) so that they lie alongside the temporal lobe.

Frontal lobe The part of the brain associated with personality and behaviour. Seizures in the frontal lobe are usually very resistant to drug treatment.

Frontal lobectomy An operation to remove the part of the frontal lobe of the brain from which seizures arise.

GABA Gamma Amino Butyric Acid – the inhibitory neural messenger of the brain.

Generalized seizure A seizure which arises over a wide area of the brain, and affects both sides of the body right from the start of the seizure.

Glutamate One of the common excitatory neural messengers of the brain.

Grand mal The old term for tonic clonic seizure (q.v.).

Half-life The time it takes for the level of a drug in the blood to fall back to half its peak level. A drug with a short half-life will need to be taken more often to be effective.

Hemiplegia Weakness or paralysis on one side of the body.

Hemispherectomy An operation to remove a badly damaged half (or hemisphere) of the brain, either partly or completely.

Hyperventilation Rapid, deep breathing carried out during an EEG recording to try to stimulate abnormal brain rhythms.

Idiopathic epilepsy Epilepsy whose cause is not known.

Idiosyncratic reaction An atypical, unpredictabale response by an individual to a normal or low dose of a drug.

Infantile spasms (West's syndrome) A rare and serious form of childhood epilepsy which usually results in some degree of learning difficulty.

Jacksonian epilepsy   Another term for motor seizure (q.v.).

Juvenile myoclonic epilepsy   A common generalized epilepsy, usually starting in the teens. There may be mild involuntary jerks of the limbs, occurring first thing in the morning, for some months before the appearance of seizures.

Ketogenic diet   A diet in which most of the daily energy requirements come from animal fats and dairy products, making the body more acid. It has been found to reduce seizures in some children.

Lesionectomy   The removal of a lesion from the brain.

Magnetic Resonance Imaging (MRI)   A way of producing a detailed picture of the structure of the brain by measuring its response to a strong magnetic field.

Motor seizure   A partial seizure affecting muscles in one part of the body. It usually starts with stiffness or jerkiness of part of the face or a limb, and may then 'march' on to affect the whole limb and then the rest of the body.

Myoclonic seizures   Sudden, brief, uncontrollable muscle jerks which usually affect one side of the body or one limb, but can affect both sides, and may be violent enough to fling the person off balance.

Neurology   The study of the nervous system and its diseases. A neurologist is the medical specialist in this field.

Neurone   A nerve cell within the nervous system. There are 10^{10} neurones in the brain.

Non-epileptic seizures   Attacks which look like epileptic seizures, but do not show the abnormal brain discharges of a true epileptic seizure. They have an emotional cause, and are a piece of abnormal behaviour.

Partial seizure   A seizure which involves only one part of the brain.

Petit mal   The old term for absence seizure (q.v.).

Photosensitive epilepsy   Epilepsy in which seizures are often triggered by flickering light.

Positron Emission Tomography (PET)   Used as a method of diagnosing epilepsy by determining the blood flow throughout the brain, to show which parts of the brain are active.

Placebo An inert tablet which has no chemical effect and is often used to compare with the effects of a new drug in drug trials.

Psychotherapy Treatment by talking: the sufferer finds relief by talking about his special problems to a trained counsellor or psychotherapist, and by obtaining their support.

Psychometric tests Tests which are used to discover which part of the brain may be damaged by assessing different mental skills.

Secondary generalized seizure A partial seizure (q.v.) that spreads rapidly throughout the brain and affects the whole body.

Seizure A sudden burst of abnormal electrical activity which temporarily affects the functioning of the brain, causing a change in emotions, consciousness, intellect or behaviour.

Seizure focus A localized area of damage in the brain which gives rise to partial seizures.

Side-effects Effects (usually undesirable) which may be produced by the normal dose of a drug in addition to its desired therapeutic effect.

Simple partial seizure A seizure which involves only part of the brain and does not affect consciousness.

Single Photon Emission (Computer) Tomography (SPECT or SPET) A less accurate scanning method similar to PET but using a different radioactive chemical.

Sphenoidal EEG A special EEG procedure to record abnormal electrical activity deep in the brain, to discover the source of seizures. Wires are inserted into the cheek and lie in the muscles outside the skull, under the temporal lobe.

Spike A rapid (lasting less than 70 milliseconds) electrical discharge seen in an EEG recording and sometimes suggestive of an epileptic focus.

Spike and wave activity An EEG epilepsy pattern. If three spikes and waves are seen per second, this is characteristic of absence seizures.

Temporal lobe The area of the brain concerned with memory and emotions, and on the left side, with some speech. Because it is easily damaged by lack of oxygen, it is often the source of epileptic activity.

Temporal lobe epilepsy   A form of epilepsy which arises in one of the temporal lobes of the brain and usually results in complex partial seizures.

Temporal lobectomy   An operation to remove the part of the temporal lobe of the brain from which seizures arise.

Todd's paralysis   Weakness affecting a limb for some hours after a motor seizure.

Tonic clonic seizure   A seizure in which there is first a violent contraction of the muscles (the tonic phase), followed by a clonic phase in which the muscles jerk in unison.

Toxic side-effects   Undesirable effects of a drug which develop if too high a dose is given.

Tuberous sclerosis   A genetically inherited type of epilepsy, also known as Bourneville's disease.

Video monitoring   Simultaneous video and EEG recording of a seizure, carried out so that changes in behaviour can be correlated with changes in EEG activity.

USEFUL ADDRESSES

British Epilepsy Association
Anstey House
40 Hanover Square
Leeds LS3 1BE

0113 2439393
Freephone Helpline: 0800 309030

The British Epilepsy Association has a network of about 150 voluntarily-run support branches, which normally meet once a month. Branches give support and information to people with epilepsy, their families and friends, and organize local advice and information events, fund-raising events and occasional social events. If you would like to know if there is a branch in your area contact the Helpline (Monday–Thursday 9.00 a.m. to 4.30 p.m., Friday 9.00 a.m. to 4.00 p.m.) and ask to speak to an Advice and Information Officer.

SPECIAL ASSESSMENT CENTRES FOR PATIENTS WITH SEVERE EPILEPSY

Bootham Park Hospital
Bootham
York YO3 7BY

Chalfont Centre for Epilepsy
Chalfont St Peter
Gerrards Cross
Buckinghamshire SL9 0RJ

01494 873 991

Maudsley Hospital Epilepsy Unit
Denmark Hill
London SE5

0171 733 6333

Ninewells Hospital
Dundee DD2 1UB

01382 660111

Radcliffe Infirmary
Oxford

01865 311188

David Lewis Centre
Warford
Nr Alderley Edge
Cheshire SK9 7UD

01565 872613

National Assessment Centre for Children with Epilepsy
Park Hospital
Old Road
Headington
Oxford OX3 7LQ

01865 245651

EPILEPSY CLINICS IN THE UK

Bootham Park Hospital
York YO3 7BY

01904 610777

Manchester Royal Infirmary
Oxford Road
Manchester M13 9WL

0161 276 1234

Walton Hospital
Rice Lane
Liverpool L9 1AE

0151 525 3611

The National Hospital
Queen Square
London WC1N 3BG

0171 837 361

The University Hospital of Wales
Heath Park
Cardiff CF4 4XW

01222 747747

Doncaster Royal Infirmary Epilepsy Clinic
Doncaster DN2 5LT

01302 366666

Queen Elizabeth Hospital
Mindelsohn Way
Edgbaston
Birmingham B15 2TH

0121 472 1311

Burden Neurological Hospital
Stapleton
Bristol BS16 1QT

0117 9567444

HOSPITALS/CENTRES FOR CHILDREN WITH EPILEPSY

Royal Manchester Children's Hospital
Hospital Road
Pendlebury
Manchester M27 1HA

0161 794 4696

Royal Preston Hospital
Sharoe Green Lane North
Fillwood
Preston PR2 4HT

01772 71565

Park Hospital for Children
Old Road
Headington
Oxford OX3 7LQ

01865 245651

Royal Liverpool Children's Hospital
Myrtle Street
Liverpool L12 2AP

0151 228 4811

University Hospital of Wales
Heath Park
Cardiff CF4 4XW

01222 755944

SPECIAL SCHOOLS FOR CHILDREN WITH EPILEPSY

David Lewis Centre
Warford
Nr. Alderley Edge
Cheshire SK9 6PW

01565 872613

St. Piers Lingfield
St. Piers Land
Lingfield
Surrey

01342 832243

St. Elizabeth's School
Much Hadham
Herts SG10 6EW

01279 843451

RESIDENTIAL HOMES FOR PEOPLE WITH EPILEPSY

David Lewis Centre
Warford
Nr. Alderley Edge
Cheshire SK9 7UD

01565 872613

St. Elizabeth's Home (women aged 16–45)
Much Hadham
Herts SG10 6EW

01279 843451

Meath Home (women)
Westbrook Road
Godalming
Surrey GU7 2QJ

01483 426162

The Maghull Homes
Liverpool Road South
Maghull
Merseyside L31 8BR

0151 526 4133

INDEX

ABC charts 97–100
absence seizure *see* seizure, absence
acupuncture 90
acetazolamine (diamox), *see* drugs
adolescent with epilepsy 161–72
alcohol 122–4
anxiety 163
aromatherapy 89
attitudes 112–3
aura 11, 12, 18–9
  epigastric 12

behaviour, 'acting out' *see* anxiety
behavioural programmes 109
benzodiazepines *see* drugs
Brain 3, 4, 5, 7
  cells 6
  damage 6, 16
  sensory cortex 11
  temporal lobe 12
  tumor 16–7
breastfeeding 198
Bourneville's disease 14
bowel/bladder control 7

callosotomy *see* surgery
carbamazepine (tegretol) *see* drugs
catamenial epilepsy *see* epilepsy, catamenial
chart, ABC *see* ABC chart
children with epilepsy 143–72

diagnosis 144–5
febrile convulsions 158
medication 150–1
school 151–4
clobazam (frisium) *see* drugs
clonazepam (rivotril) *see drugs*
contraception 190–2
covert desensitization 85–7
CT scan *see* scan, CT

denial 164
diagnosis 4, 25–8
diazepam (valium) *see* drugs
diet 118–22
disabling conditions 181–2
  Lennox Gastuar Syndrome 181
  Landau Kleffne 181
  Rasmussen's Syndrome 181
doctor, relationship with 58–60
driving regulations 136–8
drop attacks 10
drugs used in the treatment of epilepsy:
  acetazolamine (diamox) 54
  benzodiazepines 52
  carbamezepine (tegretol) 45
  clobazam (frisium) 54
  clonazepam (rivotril) 52
  diazepam (valium) 52
  ethosuximide (zarontin) 50
  gabapentin (neurontin) 56
  lamotrigine (lamictal) 51

phenobarbitone (luminal) 54
phenytoin (epanutin) 47
primidone (mysoline) 55
sodium valprote (epilim) 48
topiramate (topramax) 57
vigabatrin (sabril) 56
dysphasia 12

electric firing discharge 4, 5, 11
electroencephalography 30–3
electroencephalogram (EEG) 5,
8, 9, 31
EEG telemetry 32–3
emergency aid 132–5
employment 139–42
opportunities 182–3
epilepsy
automatisms 20–2
catamenial 189
causes of
adult epilepsy 16
childhood epilepsy 15
febrile convulsions 16
head injury 15–6
definition of 3
motor 11
myoclonic 9
juvenile 9
photosensitive 124–6
epileptic fit 5, 133
epileptic seizures see seizures,
epileptic
epileptic personality 23
epileptic spike discharge 5
ethosuximide (zarontin) see drugs
exercise 127–9

fears
children's 146–7
parent's 157–61
febrile convulsions 155–7

fertility 190
folic acid 58
first fit 26–8
frontal lobe surgery see surgery,
frontal lobe

gabapentin (neurontin) see drugs
grand mal see seizures, tonic
clonic

happiness 116–7
hemispherectomy see surgery,
hemispherectomy
heterotopia 14
Hippocrates 3
HRT and epilepsy 192–3

infantile spasms (West's Syndrome)
10
inheritance 14
investigations 30–9

Jacksonian epilepsy 11
Jackson, Hughlings 11
JME see epilepsy, juvenile
myoclonic

lamotrigine (lamictal) see drugs
Landau Kleffne see disabling
conditions
learning disabilities in children
174–80
Lennox Gastuar Syndrome see
disabling conditions

marriage 185
medication
children 150–1
cosmetic effects 165–6
meditation 91–2
memory 15

menopause 192
menstruation and epilepsy 188–90
mental retardation 14
motor epilepsy *see* epilepsy, motor
MRI scan *see* scan, MRI
myths about epilepsy 23–4

pacemaker cells 6
paroxysmal bursts 6
parent's concerns 157–61
parent's epilepsy 129–32
partial seizure *see* seizures, partial
PET scanning 38
petit mal see seizure, absence
phenobarbitone (luminal) *see* drugs
phenytoin (epanutin) *see* drugs
photosensitive epilepsy *see* epilepsy, photosensitive
post traumatic amnesia 15
pregnancy 193–8
primidone (mysoline) *see* drugs
psychometric tests 36–8

Rasmussen's Syndrome *see* disabling conditions
relaxation 81–5
regression 163
recreational (street) drugs 166–70

safety precautions 127–9
scan, CT 33–6
    MRI 33–6
school 151–4
seizures, epileptic
    absence (*petit mal*) 8
    after a seizure 19
    conditions 4
    control of 75–102
    description of 2, 17–8

febrile convulsions 155
focal 6
generalized 7
grand mal 5
localized 6
making them happen 10–2
partial 7, 10–2, 16
tonic clonic (*grand mal*) 6, 7, 8, 9, 13
triggers 17, 108–9
warnings 18–9
seizures, non-epileptic 103–110
sex 186
sex drive 171
    lack of 186–7
    fear of seizures during sex 187
sexual development 171
sodium valproate (epilim) *see* drugs
specialists, referral to 29–30
sport 127–9
status epilepticus 22
stress 163
stroke 17
surgery 62
    callosotomy 73
    hemispherectomy 71–2
    temporal lobe 66–70
    frontal lobe 70–1

temporal lobe surgery, *see* surgery, temporal lobe
Todd's paralysis 11
treatment of epilepsy 40–61
tuberous sclerosis (Bourneville's disease) 14
tonic clonic convulsions (grand mal) *see* seizures, tonic clonic
topiramate (topramax) *see* drugs
trigger situations *see* seizures, triggers

VDUs 125–6
vigabatrin (sabril) *see* drugs
video games 126
videorecording 88

warnings 18–9
women and epilepsy 188–99
wonder drugs 57

Yoga 92